Notice to the Reader:

The information contained in this book is for educational purposes only. It is not intended to be used to diagnose any ailment or prescribe any remedy. It is not meant to be a substitute for professional help. It is intended to set forth historical uses of natural remedies. A person should consult a duly approved health professional for any condition which requires their services. This information is not intended as a substitute for qualified medical care.

Neither the author nor the publisher directly or indirectly dispenses medical advice or prescribes the use of natural remedies as a form of treatment. The author and publisher disclaim any liability if the reader uses or prescribes any remedies, natural or otherwise, for him/herself or for another.

Table of Contents

Introduction

TRADITIONAL AND MODERN MEDICINE

Throughout history, man has been plagued by illness, deformities, and discomfort. And from the beginning of time, man has sought relief from these problems. Over time and through experience many different techniques and methods have been used in an effort to live a healthy life. Human beings used whatever materials were available to them. Trial and error were used to test the effectiveness. Different methods experimented with included plants, manipulation, spiritual healing, massage, and even mystical chanting. And over time, successful methods were found which enabled people to treat many ills using natural methods.

MODERN MEDICINE

Modern medicine departed from the traditional methods proven in the past. It has opted for synthetic drug intervention and immediate surgery to cure the ills we face. In fact, the traditional methods used in the past are ridiculed by some members of the modern medical community.

NATURAL MEDICINE BECOMING MORE ACCEPTED

But times are changing. More and more people are looking for alternative methods for treatment of their ailments. And the medical community is aware of this change. Many medical doctors are incorporating the use of these natural therapies in their practices. And the population seems to appreciate their efforts. The natural approach seems to be coming back into vogue. People appreciate an alternative to synthetic drug therapies that often have debilitating side effects while concentrating on only the symptoms associated with an illness. Modern health practices seem to have taken a step backwards toward "folk remedies." In reality, natural medicine is merely the return to the center of the pendulum of medicine which had swung too far towards technology and is now returning to the natural.

The Miracle of Modern Medicine

Modern medicine offers tremendous benefits to us as patients. Many modern instruments and drug therapies deserve the label miracle that has been placed upon them.

Unfortunately, the success of modern medicine often dazzles us into believing that it is the only way. And we are unable to appreciate the limitations associated with modern practices.

Modern scientific methods require two factors in order to devise a cure:

1. An identifiable condition, and
2. A condition independent of other circumstances.

Limitations on Modern Medicine

Only when these conditions are present can the modern research physician test various cures. When stated in these terms, the limitations of this approach are obvious. No condition in the body, especially disease, is independent of the rest of the body. The available modern medical treatments are limited to those which are reactive in nature and which treat independently discernable afflictions.

Holistic Approach

The natural health movement approaches these situations differently.

The natural health practitioners believe that prevention is the most practical approach to healthy living. If you feel fine, your doctor can do nothing for you. Come back when you are sick. Modern medicine takes the position that one must react to disease, find the cause of a problem and treat it. This narrow approach allows the physician the opportunity to track cures and results and pronounce certain cures as effective and others ineffective. Natural medicine looks at the individual as a whole and treats the body as a whole. The holistic approach involves keeping the body healthy and avoiding a problem before it occurs. They offer natural methods derived from natural sources as opposed to the synthesized medicines.

Nature and our Bodies

Natural health advocates offer a whole body (holistic) approach. The body is related to mother earth and our environment in many more ways than we can imagine. In order to live in better harmony with nature, we should take advantage of the beneficial things of the earth.

Nature in Modern Medicine

Modern medical research is heading out of the lab and into the wilderness. Cancer researchers have recently stated their efforts to look for cures in the rain forests. They are looking at local folklore throughout the world to search for clues to cures. A recent movie starring Sean Connery entitled "Medicine Man" depicted a doctor searching for a cure for cancer. And maybe they were on the right track. There are immense possibilities in the plant kingdom. And many drugs are based on plant research and use even now. More work is being encouraged using natural methods.

Our Environment and Health

Man has always been dependent on nature and the environment. Trying to control these leads many cultures to look for help in the mystical and supernatural. Early civilizations looked at disease as a punishment for some sin and sought to cleanse the soul of the individual. We are still very dependent on our environments.

Unfortunately our world is not perfect. And we are subjected to the effects of our own misuse of the world in which we live. Toxins are all around. Opulance has brought with it cases of heart disease, obesity, cancer, high blood pressure, as well as other illnesses. Our water and food supply are full of pesticides and pollution. And toxic metals are thought of as a major health hazard. And even exposure to the sun is becoming risky because of the depletion of the ozone layer due to pollution.

The Theory of Natural Health

The natural approach is thought to help rid the body of these toxic factors and aid in building and strengthening the body. The emphasis is on taking charge of our own health and prevention. The alternative medicine movement attracts more and more followers daily. While it was once the home for "earth-children," its appeal is becoming more broad based. Simply speaking, today's natural health means recognizing the important relationship between what we do to our bodies and our health.

The purpose of this book is not to focus on treatment of disease, although some treatments are discussed. Rather, this book is designed to reveal a healthy lifestyle intended to aid in the prevention of disease, so that remedies whether natural or synthetic will not be required as frequently and will be responded to more fully by the body.

Prevention V. Cure

The common medical practice deals with curing the problems as they occur. And often this means relieving symptoms but neglecting the cause of the problem. Andrew Weil, M.D. summarizes his view on prevention in his book entitled, NATURAL HEALTH, NATURAL MEDICINE, published by Houghton Mifflin Company, 1990. On page vii he states, "timely and appropriate investment of energy in your well-being will save a great deal of trouble, pain, and money down the road. Many people understand the value of preventive maintenance in caring for their cars. They get regular oil changes and tune-ups, and they pay attention when a warning light comes on. It is strange that more of us do not apply the same concept to our bodies, which are infinitely more valuable."

Dr. Weil makes a valid point. It is important to think of prevention first. We should keep our bodies in the best condition possible to best avoid illness. We need to be concerned and to take responsibility for our own health. This includes proper diet, exercise, health maintenance, and emotional stability. Our bodies are a whole and every aspect needs to be taken care of and maintained.

A Chinese proverb summarizes prevention. "The superior doctor prevents sickness; The mediocre doctor attends to impending sickness; The inferior doctor treats actual sickness." The natural approach focuses on maintaining the health and vigor of the patients. And the Chinese still follow this path.

Balance

The concept of balance in a person's life is perhaps the most important healthful living principle. Proper balance means adjusting ones lifestyle so that the body can tend to its own needs. Three elements that go into this balance are diet, exercise and lifestyle. The proper balance does not mean that one will avoid all disease. But rather that the body will better be able to resist disease and and fight it if attacked.

We are all searching for a balance in life. Many adhere strictly to the natural methods, while others consider the natural to be unhealthy, unsafe, and pure quackery.

Balance in life implies both internal balance among the various body parts and systems and external balance with the environment in which we live. True balance seems to be in living in harmony with our own bodies as well as our environment. Conflict within ourselves or between us and our environment is the antithesis of balance.

Just as the natural approach has a place, so does the medical community. It is important to remember that many acute and life-threatening situations require immediate results. Generally the natural approach requires a longer period of time to work. The natural method works on cleaning the body and helping the body heal itself while the conventional medical technique usually concentrates on relieving immediate symptoms.

Natural medicine is not intended to replace modern medicine. However, it should not be dismissed or ignored because it does not depend on modern technology or because its benefits are not readily discernable in a controlled environment. Natural medicine should be appreciated for its ability to help individuals enjoy a higher quality of life

Natural Health for Today's Lifestyles

But many of the natural or holistic health books available on the market today assume that the reader will turn over his/her life to these new methods. In reality, most people are more interested in taking steps toward natural health. They don't have the interest in going completely natural but may like to adapt some methods to bring their lives closer into balance with nature. This book will serve as an introduction to natural health; a primer for the less than fully committed; a manual for the nineties for people on the go.

This book will serve as a method of introducing the basic, well-known principles involved with natural or holistic approaches to health. It will discuss achieving balance in life, proper diet, exercise and introduce natural health supplements.

THE THEORY OF NATURAL HEALTH

Introduction to Traditional Medicine

TRADITIONAL REMEDIES

Herbology

The use of the healing properties of plants is the oldest of the traditional remedies. Today it is often difficult to draw a line between the herbalist and the medical doctor because of the extensive use of plants and plant extracts in modern medicines.

HERBS USED ANCIENTLY

The plant kingdom has always provided people with food and medicine. References to the use of medicinal herbs are found throughout the Bible. All ancient cultures used them. Herbs were thought to be magical and full of healing benefits. Today herbs are used throughout the world to provide treatment, especially in many developing countries and throughout Western Europe and the Far East.

HERBS USED TODAY

Folklore was the traditional method for learning herbal remedies and treatments. This knowledge of how to heal and maintain health was passed down to each generation. Families shared their knowledge with neighbors. They took care of each other. They relied on the earth to provide the materials necessary to treat ailments.

A Natural Method

Herbs are a natural means of providing the body with essential nutrients to aid in the healing process. Herbs feed the body just as food does, and they work with the body to help strengthen and build it up as it heals itself. Herbalists believe that the body can heal itself using natural herbal therapy to activate and support the body's own self-healing powers.

Herbs contain many nutritious elements. They are most effective when they are not refined or synthesized but are used in their natural, balanced state. Herbalists believe that the body is able to receive and assimilate the nutrients it requires. It is able to utilize these herbs where they are needed in the body at any particular time.

Different From Drugs

Herbs work differently than drugs made from plants. Drugs usually contain a single active substance which has been extracted from a plant or synthesized. Herbs, on the other hand, provide a broad array of catalysts which work together harmoniously to provide the body with a complete healing network. Instead of focusing on an isolated segment of a body system, herbs work with the whole system. Herbalists believe that the natural approach to health using herbs can add health and vigor to the body.

Time Required to Heal

Generally, the actions of herbs require a period of time to be effective. Their action is subtle. This method is usually gradual. In fact, slow healing major health problems are thought to allow time for the body to heal itself throughout. Herbalists agree that this slow, natural approach is ultimately more effective in offering a permanent cure to an ailment. Individuals who have chosen to abuse their bodies for many years may take even longer to see changes from herbal remedies. Using herbal treatments requires one to stop what they are doing and slow down.

Side Effects of Drugs

Drugs made synthetically or extracted from plants are not used in their natural form. People are finding that often the side effects of drugs cause more problems than the drugs alleviate. Drugs are often called chemicals because the compounds are taken from a natural state and synthesized and made into an unnatural state. Herbs generally contain natural buffers and synergistic substances which help balance and make the herb more useful. Drugs are often taken in a form that is foreign to the body and may disrupt its internal harmony. Herbalists feel that this is the reason for side effects associated with many prescribed and over-the-counter drugs.

Drugs are a result of the fast paced world in which we live and our modern refusal to take responsibility for our actions. We want an immediate cure to a problem. We want the doctor to prescribe a pill to rid us of the symptoms that afflict our bodies without being willing to look to ourselves as the cause of our own problem and without changing our diet or lifestyle. The medical community responds and often treats the problem, neglecting the cause of the condition. The natural approach is to look at the cause while working on healing the whole body rather than only treating the symptoms of an illness.

Emergencies

Yet modern herbalists do not abandon modern medicine. Each has its place. In a life threatening situation, it is important to remember that any method capable of saving a life should be used. Emergencies require immediate results. There is certainly a place for the medical community in this world in which we live. Herbalists believe that the natural methods can coexist with the modern medical therapies.

Herbs Treat Whole Systems

Herbs, as with other foods, need to be used with wisdom and knowledge. Different herbs are used to help different problems. Individual herbs and herbal combinations can be found for every system of the body. Some herbs benefit the nervous system, others the digestive system, and still others the circulatory, glandular, immune, respiratory, intestinal, urinary and the skeletal and muscular systems. Modern research has added much knowledge about the effectiveness of these herbal remedies. They are believed to contain properties which can heal and build the body. Herbs are known to be rich in vitamins and minerals which work with the body to heal specific areas.

Books Help With Research

Reputable herbalists rely on study and research to determine the effectiveness of individual herbs and of combinations of herbs. There are many books on the market offering advice and information of uses and ways in which these herbal remedies can and should be used. And many of these books have been written by medical doctors who choose to use this natural method whenever possible. The bibliography lists a number of useful herb books.

Methods of Application

Herbs are available and used in many forms. Some individuals prefer to grow and cultivate their own herbal gardens. Others purchase the herbs in many forms which include teas, capsules, ointments, compresses, extracts, oils, poultices, powders, salves, syrups, and tinctures.

Teas or Infusions

The most common use of herbs is in the form of an infusion or tea. This is made by pouring hot liquid over the herb and steeping. The ratio recommended is usually 1/2 to 1 oz. of herb to 1 pint of water. Enamel, porcelain or glass pots are suggested. They should steep for 10 to 20 minutes and then be covered with a tight lid to avoid evaporation. The tea should be strained into a cup before drinking. Generally the teas should be taken lukewarm or cold. To induce sweating or break up congestion, they may be taken hot.

Capsules

Gelatin capsules provide an easy and pleasant method of taking herbs, especially those that are bitter tasting. When purchased from a quality company, the herbs can be depended upon to be clean and combined in correct proportions. They are usually prepared and measured by chemists trained in the herbs. Capsules should be taken with a large glass of water or herbal tea to help them dissolve.

Ointments

Ointments are used on the skin when the active principles of herbs are needed for extended periods to accelerate healing. They are usually used in cases of injury, contusion and effusion. Some vaseline products made from natural sources can be used instead of petroleum products. One or two heaping tablespoons of the herb or herbs are brought to boil in the vaseline. The mixture is then stirred or strained. When cold, the ointment is put into jars.

Compresses

An herbal compress is used to produce similar effects as an ointment but using heat. One or two heaping tablespoons of the herb are boiled in one cup of water. A sterile cotton pad or gauze is dipped in the strained liquid and placed on the affected area while still warm. It can then be covered with a woolen material.

Small children should have it bandaged into place. When cold, the compress should be changed. This method is usually used in cases of injury, contusions, and effusions. It is also used when herbs may be too strong to be taken internally and allows them to be absorbed in small amounts.

Decoction

A decoction is a method of preparing herbs when a plant is not readily soluble in cold or hot water, but it becomes soluble when boiled and simmered in water for five to twenty minutes. Five minutes is usually enough for finely shredded material. If the herb is hard or woody, twenty minutes may be necessary. It usually works best if the plant is soaked in cold water first and then brought to a boil. A teaspoon of dried herb is placed in an enamel or glass container with one cup of pure water. Decoctions should be strained while they are hot. This method is thought to be valuable for extracting mineral salts and alkaloids from the herbs. A decoction should generally be used within 24 hours of preparation.

Extracts

Herbal extracts are rubbed into the skin for treating strained muscles and ligaments, arthritis, or inflammation. They usually contain stimulating herbs such as cayenne and lobelia. An extract can be made by putting four ounces of dried herbs or eight ounces of fresh bruised herbs into a jar. Add one pint of vinegar, alcohol or massage oil and allow to sit. The jar should be shaken once or twice daily. It takes about four days for powdered herbs and 15 days for whole or cut herbs. Extracts can also be purchased from health food stores or professional herb companies.

Oils

Herb oils are useful when ointments or compresses are not practical. Oils are prepared by pounding the fresh or dried herbs. Olive oil or sesame oil is added and the mixture is put in a warm place for about four days. (2 oz. of herb to one pint of oil) Another method is to heat the oil in a pan for one hour for use sooner. The oil is strained and bottled. A small amount of vitamin E is usually added to help preserve the preparation. Oils are usually made from the aromatic herbs such as eucalyptus, peppermint, spearmint and spices. The oils should be stored in dark glass bottles for greater shelf life.

POULTICES

A poultice is a warm mashed-fresh or ground and powdered herb applied directly to the skin to relieve inflammation, blood poisoning, venomous bites, boils, abscess, or to cleanse and heal an affected area. The skin should be oiled before applying the hot poultice. The herb can be mixed with water or another liquid to form a paste. The poultice should be covered with a clean cloth when applied to the affected area.

POWDERS

Powders are made from fresh plant parts and mashed until there are fine particles of the herbal agent. They can be taken in capsules, herbal teas, water or sprinkled in food.

SALVES

Fresh or dried herbs are covered with water, brought to a boil, and simmered for thirty minutes. The herbs are then strained and added to an equal amount of olive or safflower oil. It is simmered until the water has evaporated into steam and only the oil is left. Beeswax can be added to give the mixture a salve consistency. It should be stored in a dark glass jar with a tight lid.

SYRUPS

Herbs in a syrup base are used for treating coughs, congestion, and throat problems. They coat and soothe the affected area. Syrups are made by adding about two ounces of herbs to a quart of water and gently boiling down to one pint. Honey and or glycerine can be added for flavor. Licorice and wild cherry bark are commonly used as flavorings.

TINCTURES

Tinctures are solutions of concentrated herbal extracts that can be kept for long periods of time. Alcohol is often added as a preservative. Tinctures are useful for herbs that do not taste good or are to be taken over an extended period of time. They may also be used externally as a liniment.

Tinctures are generally used with more potent herbs that are usually not used as herbal teas. They can be made by combining four ounces of powdered or cut herb with one pint of alcohol such as vodka, brandy, gin or rum. It should be shaken daily and let sit for two weeks. The herbs should settle and the tincture can be poured off. The powder should be strained out with cheese cloth. They can also be made using vinegar.

Aromatherapy

THE USE OF SCENTS

Aromatherapy is the practice of using scents to influence moods and pain and to treat and cure minor ailments. The theory of Aromatherapy is based upon the fact that the olfactory and emotional centers of the body are connected. And that by inhaling different aromas, emotional concerns as well as physical complaints can be eased. This form of natural treatment is related to the use of herbs but relies on the benefits of the oils of the plants.

SMELL AND HEALING

The nose is responsible for identifying odors. Smells are related to how we perceive and remember the world and events. Certain odors bring out memories of the past. For this reason, the sense of smell is thought to be involved in the memory function of the brain. And it is also used to identify problems in the body such as infection.

HISTORICAL USES OF AROMATICS

Historically, the Egyptians used aromatics in the mummification process: myrrh, frankincense, cedarwood and cassia oils. The Hebrews, on the other hand, used them for special purification rituals. In the Song of Solomon, spikenard, saffron, calamus, cinnamon, frankincense, myrrh, aloes, lily, and camphire are mentioned. The book of John in the Bible relates the incident in which Mary anointed the feet of Christ with spikenard, filling the room with the odor of the ointment. The Greeks considered aromatic plants gifts from the gods. The Romans used scented oils and perfumes by adding them to their famous baths in Rome and Pompeii. Avicenna, the famous Arabian doctor of the tenth century, was the first to use the process of distillation for essential oils. In the Middle Ages bags of strong smelling herbs were carried by many.

THE FOUNDING OF THE PERFUME

And Essential oils probably began the perfume industry. The practice of aromatherapy has been around for thousands of years and continues to be used today.

HISTORY OF AROMATHERAPY

The title aromatherapy is credited to Rene Maurice Gatlefosse, a French cosmetic chemist and was introduced about twenty years ago. His theory is that the essential oils can help the skin and help heal dermatitis. These oils can also help with infections and work as a natural antibiotic. A colleague of Gatlefosse, Godissart, later began an aromatherapy clinic in the United States treating skin cancer, gangrene, osteomalacia and facial ulcers with lavender oil. To him the most important aspect was for the patient to have an actual perception of the fragrance and its usefulness. Dr. Paolo Rovesti of Milan University in Italy studied the effects essential oils have on the mind. He sprayed these essences around patients and found that this therapy served as nerve stimulants or sedatives to treat depression and anxiety.

Modern Use of Aromatics

This type of therapy is becoming more popular in the United States. And as people look for alternative methods of treatment, some are finding the answer in the use of aromatherapy. Elizabeth Arden and Estee Lauder, who are two well know names in the cosmetic industry, are introducing lines of Sensory Therapy products. And even the airline industry is getting into the practice. They are using some products known as After Flight Regulator oils. The July 1, 1992, issue of the USA Today newspaper printed an article on Aromatherapy. It noted that "Dr. Robert Henkin of the Taste and Smell Clinic in Washington, D.C., believes aromatherapy is blossoming now because "people are becoming more aware in the '90s that natural things have natural consequences." He says aromatherapy is already in our daily lives, in scented soaps and bath oils and cooking spices. The amount of essential oils sold in the U.S. increased by 102.6 million ounces over the past two years, according to the Fragrance Materials Association. Sales are up $18 million over that period."

Plant Sources

The essential oils are all considered to be natural substances. They are a part of the plant but also separate from the other compositions of the plant. The essence of the plants is thought to have similar properties to that plant but it also is more subtle and more connected to emotions.

Preparation

The essential oils are found in very small amounts in plants. They are removed from the plants by various methods including pressing, distillation, tapping, and separation using heat. Most of the essential oils are colorless. But some have color such as cinnamon which is has a reddish tone. The essences are found in the plants. But some aromas in some plants are only formed with water.

DIFFERENT ESSENCES

The essences found in plants are complicated substances. They contain many different compounds. They are divided into three categories:

1. Hydrocarbon essences (the largest category)
2. Oxygenized essences
3. Sulphurized essences

NATURAL OILS

These essences are sometimes copied in synthetic forms, but these are not thought to be as effective as the natural substance. Aromatherapy is thought to be the most effective when using the original form of the oil. A synthetic oil is not thought to contain the life force of the plant. The actual structure of the plant cannot be duplicated. The odors can sometimes be duplicated to a certain extent, but they are not considered to be as therapeutic for the body.

EXTERNAL APPLICATION

The essences are usually applied externally. This allows the essence to travel through the skin to the body fluids resulting in the gradual absorption in the body. The oils affect different areas of the body through the blood and body fluids.

SMALL DOSAGES

Aromatherapy is similar to homeopathy in that the doses are generally given in small amounts. This is thought to be the most effective method of administration.

The essential oils need to be kept in sealed, colored, glass containers to protect them from the air and light.

Aromatherapy includes massaging the essential oils into the body. This is considered to aid in relieving tension and improving circulation.

Basic Oils

The following are some of the basic oils that are readily available:

Orange Oil: This is thought to aid in relieving tension and relaxing the body.

Spearmint Oil: This is recommended for use with stomach problems. It can aid digestion and help relieve nausea.

Peppermint Oil: This essence is used in cases of fever, headache and to increase energy in the body.

Eucalyptus Oil: This is often used with problems associated with colds and allergies. It is used for sinus complaints and is effective in relieving a stuffy nose. It is also considered beneficial in helping alleviate the pain of a sore throat.

Rose Oil: This is probably the most expensive oil. It takes approximately one hundred pounds of petals to extract 1/2 ounce of oil. Aromatherapists recommend this for digestion, headaches, and inflammation.

Rosemary Oil: This oil is taken from the flowering tops of the plant. It is used for digestion, scalp problems, relaxation, memory aid, and circulation.

Chamomile Oil: This oil is refreshing with a fruity odor. It is used as a general tonic and is soothing on the body and mind.

Lavender Oil: English lavender is considered to be the best. It is used to promote a restful sleep. It should be used only in small quantities because of its strong aroma.

Jasmine Oil: This is used to aid coughs and problems of the female organs. It can be massaged into the lower back to ease the pain from cramps.

Cinnamon Oil: This oil is known for its stimulation and warmth properties. It can be massaged to increase temperature and promote warmth.

STARTING TO GROW IN U.S.

Aromatherapists are convinced that this technique can have wonderful results. Many claim fantastic results. But it is just now beginning to find popularity in the United States.

Reflexology

THEORY OF REFLEXOLOGY

Reflexology is based on the premise that the feet and the hands contain pressure points that correspond to different body parts, organs, and glands. These pressure points are connected to those specific body parts through the nervous system. By massaging specific areas on the feet and hands, stress in the corresponding area in the body can be relieved. This procedure is administered with a specific method using the thumb and fingers. When circulation in the feet is inhibited due to illness, shoes, or little exercise, deposits form at the nerve endings. Reflexologists attempt to loosen the deposits through foot massage thus encouraging the whole body to perform more effectively. Reflexology is used to relieve stress, improve circulation, and to help normalize and regain balance in the body.

ORIGINATED IN ORIENT

The Oriental culture is thought to have begun the use of reflexology nearly two thousand years ago. They associated certain circulation paths throughout the body with the feet.

They studied the effect of body parts on massage and learned to remove blockage and resume circulation.

Reflex Points

Reflexology specifically uses ten zones in the body which correspond to "reflex" points.

A reflex is an involuntary response to some form of stimulus. The organs of the body are examples of involuntary actions. They are stimulated by energy flowing through the body from the brain. If the circulation is stopped or strained, the energy flow is disrupted to the glands, organs, and muscles. The nervous system passes the messages to different points in the body. These are sent from the brain and influenced by impulses received from different stimuli. When a problems arises due to tension on a vital nerve, the whole system can suffer.

Importance of Nervous System

The blood and nerve systems are essential to the proper function of all organs and glands. The entire body works together and the nerves must be sending the correct signals efficiently to keep everything in order. As the tension eases, the nerves and vessels are able to relax allowing the flow of blood and nerve impulses to improve their function. Reflexology stresses massage and removing the blockage to allow the energy flow to continue and the body to function properly.

The system of reflexology is learned by studying books, observing, and practice. There are thought to be 72,000 nerve endings in the feet which correspond to areas of the body.

Autonomic Nervous System

Reflexology generally deals with the autonomic nervous system. There are many different types of reflexes. The autonomic reflex is thought of as involuntary. These include gland and organ function. They are activities that go on in the body without the individual really being aware or consciously controlling them. The impulses in the autonomic nervous system run vertically from the feet through the body.

FEET DETERMINE HEALTH

Reflexologists believe that the feet can determine the health of the entire body, just as iridologist believe the eyes can determine the health of the body. They feel that keeping the feet in good condition can help the body stay healthy and strong. The practice of reflexology has found its way to the western world. Many are finding relief from stress related illness through this practice.

Homeopathy

THEORY OF HOMEOPATHY

Homeopathy is the use of remedies derived from herbs, minerals and other natural substances to treat illness and disease. The theory stresses that the body takes great steps to heal itself. But sometimes an extra boost is needed. This is when homeopathic medicine in very diluted amounts can help the body to free itself of disease. Conventional treatments suppress symptoms and are sometimes temporary. For instance, antibiotics can kill harmful bacteria but they also kill the good bacteria which can leave the body susceptible to other illness.

ORIGINS OF HOMEOPATHY

The modern practice of homeopathy began in the late 1700's or early 1800's. Dr. Samuel Hahnemann, a German physician, is credited with its development. But anciently homeopathy was used in the Eastern culture and may date back as far as 3000 B.C.

Hahnemann, while experimenting with medicines, discovered that overdoses of the drug quinine in a healthy individual caused symptoms very similar to malaria. Quinine was known to cure malaria. This lead him to study the effects of giving patients drugs which normally cause the problems they were experiencing.

Theory of Similars

Hahnemann experimented on himself and others. He discovered that diluted and safe amounts of drugs that produce symptoms of a disease in a healthy person could help cure the disease without dangerous side effects. This lead him to the theory of the law of similars: Similia similibus curentur, (Let likes be cured with likes).

The law of similars states that any substance which can cause symptoms of an illness when given to a healthy person, can heal an individual who is suffering from similar symptoms. The theory is that the same anatomy of the cure and the illness are brought together to heal.

The Use of Similars In Medicine

Conventional medicine has also practiced the law of similars. In immunizations, small amounts of the disease are given to immunize a patient against that disease. Allergy sufferers are often given injections with small dilutions of the substance they react to in order to build up a tolerance. Cancer patients are given radiation treatments and radiation is known to cause cancer. These modern common medical practices are similar to the ancient homeopathy. But they do not obey the major principle of homeopathy which requires the treatment of the person as a whole physically and psychologically using one single medicine.

In homeopathy only one medicine is given at a time. Even though there may be many symptoms, homeopathic doctors feel there should be only one cure. Whether the condition be chronic or acute, one medicine should stimulate the body into action. While using just one medication the effect of the treatment can be monitored and changed more easily if necessary.

USE OF SMALL AMOUNTS

Homeopathic remedies are usually extremely diluted amounts of the original substance. The substances are usually mixed with distilled water or alcohol. The substances are shaken and diluted sometimes to a dilution of 1 in 1,000,000 parts. But the remedies are still effective in extremely diluted dosages. The phenomenon which accompanies this practice is not easily explained. It seems that some influence of the substance does remain. Homeopaths feel that there is still some force of nature or energy present in the diluted forms that can aid in curing an ailment. They feel that the remedies can help bring balance back to allow the body to function properly. They consider the remedies to work with nature and the body.

THE IMMUNE SYSTEM

Homeopaths work in concert with the body's immune system. Disease can only occur when the cause (virus, bacteria, etc.) is present and the body is susceptible to that cause because the immune system is weakened. A remedy is sought which can cause reactions similar to the symptoms associated with the disease. This is thought to alleviate the disturbance which is wrecking havoc in the body by strengthening the immune system

ACUTE AND CHONIC DISEASE

Disease is considered acute or chronic. Acute is associated with those illnesses that may be brief and end after they have run their course. Chronic illness is thought to be more destructive. It is a condition that persists over a prolonged period of time. It may flair up occasionally and gradually worsen. With chronic conditions, the homeopath must look at the whole problem discovering the origin of the disease. And then he may discover a weakness that is causing the problem and concentrate on remedies for that cause.

With some of the remedies, the symptoms may first increase before they begin to decrease. This is thought to be caused by the strengthening of the vital force or energy. In some cases it takes more than one treatment or remedy to cure an ailment. Only one remedy is administered at a time in order to monitor the results and determine necessary treatment.

Look at Symptoms

Homeopaths look at the symptoms to identify a cure. In other natural medical fields this is not the case. But the homeopath looks at the symptoms and decides a treatment. The symptoms are the means of choosing a remedy. Homeopathy seeks to find a cure before greater problems occur. Treatment occurs in the beginning when there may be only mild symptoms present.

The remedies need to be handled carefully. They can be destroyed by the exposure to sunlight, heat, or cold. They should be stored in moderate temperatures away from direct sun.

The Royal Homeopath

Homeopathy is now becoming more accepted in the western world. Western Europe has been very receptive to homeopathy. The Royal family in England are well known users of homeopathic medicine. Queen Elizabeth has her own personal homeopathic physician on her medical staff. Homeopathy is widely used in the Hindu religion and throughout India.

The U.S. has been less receptive of homeopathy. But more medical doctors are using homeopathic medicine along with traditional treatment. There seems to be an awakening of homeopathic medicine in America, and it is finding a place in the medical community.

Acupuncture

ANCIENT CHINESE PRACTICE

The practice of acupuncture dates back 4500 years. It is an ancient Chinese practice of relieving pain and treating disease by inserting needles into certain areas of the body. The Chinese believe that pain and disease are the product of an imbalance of forces in the body known as yin and yang. They use acupuncture to restore the balance.

ACUPUNCTURE POINTS

Acupuncture involves penetrating sharp needles beneath the skin to reach nerve endings that control pain. The needles are inserted into any one of hundreds of points along what acupuncturists consider the 12 paired and 2 unpaired meridians or channels of energy that run along the body. The needles are very thin. This procedure should only be done by individuals skilled and practiced in the field.

Most participants do not feel discomfort during the acupuncture procedure. But there is usually a pinching feeling that is followed by a numbness or soreness during the time the needles are in place.

THEORIES HOW ACCUPUNCTURE WORKS

Some scientists believe that acupuncture works by increasing the brain's production of the natural painkillers known as endorphins. They function similar to morphine. Another theory is that the needles inserted interrupt the pain signals through the nervous system. And in the west it is used mainly for pain management. Acupuncture is also used to aid recovering addicts with cravings and to help others with anxiety, sleep problems, and mood swings. Many rehabilitation facilities use this technique.

The Chinese have used the procedure of acupuncture to treat all types of conditions including arthritis, migraines, insomnia, ulcers, and mental illness. Some doctors in China have even used acupuncture to alleviate pain during surgery instead of anesthetics. The patients have been known to do very well and felt no pain.

Scientific evidence supporting the usefulness of acupuncture is sketchy. Yet some swear by the procedure and have documented fantastic results.

Breathing Therapy

The importance of adequate air is known to every living person. But there seem to be certain techniques of breathing that can improve the body's ability to breath. Breathing is an autonomic response as well as a voluntary action. So better breathing techniques can be learned by everyone. Deep breathing alone is important. But posture can be just as valuable. And exercise is an important ingredient in improving oxygen intake.

CONTROLLING THE BODY

Individuals involved with breathing therapy feel that learning to control the way we breath can have an effect on the involuntary functions of the body. Yoga uses this technique and many have mastered the ability to control their bodies by first learning to regulate their breathing.

BREATHING AND EMOTIONS

Breathing has connections to the emotions. Breathing changes as the moods change. An angry person may breath rapidly and shallow. Perhaps breathing can help control moods by learning to keep the breaths slow, deep, and regular.

Breathing from the diaphragm is the most effective. The diaphragm muscles push downward allowing air to be pushed into the lower lung utilizing full lung capacity. The chest then is filled with air as inhalation takes place.

A Breathing Exercise

Being aware and paying attention to breathing patterns is a key factor in improving the intake of oxygen. The following is an exercise that can be done several times each day to train yourself to utilize more fully your lung capacity:

1. Relax muscles.
2. Stand or sit with the back straight.
3. Shoulders back.
4. Exhale with a little extra push.
5. Inhale slowly through the nose while consciously filling the lungs to capacity.
6. Exhale slowly while feeling the air leave the lungs and push as much out as possible.

Exercise

Aerobic exercise can help increase the lung capacity. Regular, moderate exercise is essential to improving the body's ability to use oxygen efficiently. And aerobic exercise helps improve the fitness of the nerves and muscles that control the breathing process.

Air is essential to our existence. But unfortunately, the amount of pollution in the air is causing detrimental effects on our bodies. It increases the risk of many illnesses including respiratory diseases and those associated with a lowered immune system. Air filter systems can be purchased for the home to improve the quality of air.

Breathing techniques can be improved. By spending just a few minutes each day concentrating on breathing quality, you can train yourself to breath more efficiently.

Color Therapy

RELATIONSHIP TO LIGHT

All life is dependent upon light for existence. The changing of the seasons affects everyone. And as there is a bond between us and the sun, so there a bond between us and the colors of our world. This is the theory behind the study and practice of color therapy.

USES OF COLOR

Advertisers are aware of the effects of color. They are used to influence and hopefully entice the buyer to purchase a product. And in fact color and its influence is involved in the clothes we choose to wear, our home furnishings, and even our automobiles. There seems to be certain colors that we are the most comfortable with. Everyone has a favorite color. And children seem to be drawn to certain colors from an early age.

Some music lovers claim that they can see colors when they listen to certain musical pieces. An aria that spreads as northern lights in ice pale blue or a fugue flashing red and orange flames. Other people possess an unusual and rare demo-optical perception, having the ability to see or feel colors with their fingers. To them light colors feel smooth and thin, while dark colors are rough and heavy, yellow is slippery, soft, and light in weight. Blue is smooth and cool. Red is warm, sticky and coarse.

But light and color are thought by some to be more than just a personal preference. Some therapists suggest that color and light can affect mood and also aid in the healing process.

ORIGINAL RESEARCH

Dinshah P. Ghadiali was a leader in the research and practice of color therapy. He moved to the United States in 1911 from India where he had studied medicine. Dinshah felt that the body is made up of chemical elements. And the body also contains a balance of color and light waves. When balance in the body is off due to illness, stress, or injury, then the color waves of the body are also off balance. He felt that treatment with light and color could restore the body to a harmonic state through balancing the energy. This would restore the body and allow it to heal itself. Many believe that color therapy works to neutralize the problems that have set the body out of balance.

EINSTEIN'S PHOTOELECTRIC LAW

Albert Einstein is well known for his studies of light. Albert Einstein's Photoelectric Law explains the energy levels of different colors. Researchers noticed that when a particular wave length of light falls upon a metal plate, the plate ejects electrons at a specific velocity. If a light beam of a lower frequency strikes the plate, the electrons are ejected at reduced velocities. Only the particular color of the light, not its intensity, affects the velocity of the electrons. If the intensity of the light is diminished, fewer electrons will be ejected, but the velocity remains constant.

Although both American Indians and Egyptians used color for healing, modern practitioners insist that colors do not in themselves heal but they spark the body to perform the healing function. Colors are stimulating, depressing, peaceful or melancholy.

COLOR THERAPIES

Color therapists have utilized this process by first understanding what color is. Considering the spectrum, red has the longest wave length, while violet has the shortest. Red represents vertical and cubic; blue the horizontal and spherical; yellow, raying out and detaching. White is not a color because it is all color. It is made up of the primary colors of light, red, green and violet, and the secondary yellow and blue. Green is a neutral color and can therefore assist in any ailment.

Color therapy can be applied in the following ways.

1. Colored fabrics, walls and illumination.
2. Mental image making, counseling, guided meditation.
3. Projection to another person.

There has been a lot of research and study done on the effects of light and color. Some of the prominent researchers include John Ott, Faber Birren, Friedrich Ellinger, and Dr. Wallace F. MacNaughton. They all have done extensive research and wrote on their experiments.

Color Attributes

Examples of the effects of certain colors include:

Green

Green: Color therapists believe that green is the most important color to keep in balance. It is considered to be one of the most prominent color energies because it is responsible for taking force to the entire body. It is crisp, cool and fresh. It restores the nerves and gives energy. Green is the color everyone starts with during color therapy.

Blue

Blue: Blue is thought to be relaxing and calming. It is less hostile and stress relieving. It is also considered to have an astringent effect, helping to relieve inflammation and infection.

Yellow

Yellow: Yellow is thought to stand for creativity and inspiration. It inspires courage and self-confidence. It increases appetite, and builds nerves. It aids in sugar balance and stimulates thought.

ORANGE

Orange: This is the color of success. It stimulates and builds the lungs. It expands interest and is thought to stimulate milk production in nursing mothers.This color is associated with fatigue and is sometimes referred to as the "sun color."

RED

Red: Red is the color of aggression and tension. It is though to stimulate glandular activity, especially in the liver.

These are just a few examples. The individuals who advocate and practice light and color therapy are sure of its success. Color therapists, interior designers, doctors, psychologists and holistic doctors have found that certain colors do certain things, depending upon how they are used.

Hydrotherapy

Water is used by many as a natural therapy. It is not irritating to use internally and it is soothing to the skin. Water affects the entire body including the muscles, nerves, skin, and organs. It can help enhance and relieve fatigued and aching muscles.

A WARM BATH

Hydrotherapy uses either hot, warm, cool, or cold water. Hot or warm water dilates the blood vessels and increases the flow of blood. Local application increases capillary pressure, increases the flow of fluid into the lymph spaces, increases perspiration, and relieves pain. A warm bath relieves stress and aches and can help relax the body.

Cool or cold water slows the blood flow. When applied after an injury such as a twisted ankle, it will reduce the swelling. The cold water can deliver extra oxygen to the skin. It also gives the body new energy. A cold shower can rejuvenate and stimulate the mind and body.

HYDROTHERAPIES

Examples of some common, simple hydrotherapy techniques include:

Fomentations (warm)
- relieve congestion of chest colds
- ease pain of arthritis
- stimulate (alternate with cold)
- sedate (use on spine)

Hot foot bath (100-115 degrees)
- increase circulation
- heighten nerve and muscle tone, skin sen sitivity
- increase antibody production

Sitz bath Cold (55-75 degrees)
- hemorrhoids, prostate, perinium and rectum surgery
  Hot (105-110 degrees)
- pelvic pain during menstrual cycle, inflammatory conditions

Contrast baths (hot then cold)
- poor circulation
- arthritis

Ice packs
- injury
- swelling
- anesthetics

Tub bath neutral (94-98 degrees)

- sedative (cover the patient to the neck with a pillow under the neck)

There are many different methods of using water externally. Some include epsom salt bath, sauna, sulphur baths, and mineral baths. This is a simple technique that can achieve worthwhile results.

Chiropractics

THEORY OF CHIROPRACTICS

Chiropractors work on the premise that the spine can be the cause of disease therefore alignment of the spine by manipulation can help protect the body's vital forces. They believe that out of place vertebrae can interfere with proper nerve function. The spinal nerves are associated with all parts of the body. An out of place condition is thought to lead to some diseases by lowering the body's ability to resist illness. Chiropractors attempt to restore normal function of the nervous system and normalize the body. They use X-rays along with examinations to determine the position of vertebrae.

ITS HISTORY

The philosophy of chiropractics was introduced by Daniel David Palmer in 1895. He said that chiropractics is first a preventive form of health care and only secondly a cure. Palmer used information from Hippocrates, Plato, Aristotle, Galen and Vesalius. Hippocrates said that the spine should be watched for the cause of disease. The spinal cord is where all vital forces flow to all parts of the body.

All cells in the body receive nerve impulses either directly or indirectly from the spine.

Practitioners of Chiropractic Medicine believe that disease is caused by interference with normal nerve function. They attempt to free the body of blocked or damaged nerve control which may lessen the body's resistance to disease and infection. They believe in prevention and manipulating the spine so that the nervous system can perform its function of controlling and coordinating cells, organs, and structures in the body. The breakdown of the immune system may be avoided with the nervous system functioning properly.

Subluxations

These interferences are known as subluxations (vertebral misalignments) and are caused by birth, accidents, trauma, fear, toxins, tobacco, alcohol, fumes, and drugs. This subluxation is considered to be the main cause of disease.

Training

Chiropractors spend many hours studying the same science as medical students. They are trained in anatomy, physiology, pathology, chemistry, bacteriology, diagnosis, neurology, x-ray, psychiatry, orthopedics and gynecology. They differ in that medical students study pharmacology, immunology, and general surgery. Chiropractors study adjusting, manipulation, and kinesiology. They concentrate on improving the body so that it will be able to keep itself healthy.

Chiropractors work with the bones of the spine and skeletal system in order to free the nerves to perform their work. The bones and skeleton are keys to opening the doors to the nerves. Chiropractors are considered by some to be nerve specialists.

Most chiropractors concentrate on helping with structural problems and pain of the joints and muscles. Others choose a wide variety of problems. Generally medical doctors do not believe in the process of spinal manipulation for major problems and diseases.

Chiropractics often involves nutrition counseling. They usually follow natural approaches to health and use other methods such as hydrotherapy, herbs, massage, acupressure, and vitamin therapy along with spinal manipulation.

Charcoal Therapy

Charcoal therapy is an old fashioned remedy. It is usually used as an antidote for poisoning as well as a cleansing agent in infections and problems with the metabolic process.

ACTIVATED CHARCOAL

Activated charcoal is produced from burning wood or bone under controlled conditions. It is then treated with an oxidizing gas, such as steam of air, at elevated temperatures. The absorptive power of charcoal is enhanced with this process which actually produces fine pores in the material.

The grain of the charcoal is thought to have the ability to absorb material such as gases, foreign proteins, body wastes, chemicals, drugs, air pollutants and all foreign material in the body. It also acts as a powerful cleansing agent.

It can be used externally as well as internally for bug bites, bee stings, poison ivy, rashes or even snake bites. Some believe that the benefits of charcoal include absorbing foreign material as well as eliminating material that is not compatible with the body. It does not seem to absorb essential nutrients from the body.

Many feel that charcoal is a natural therapy that can be used safely and without reservation in healing different ailments.

USES OF CHARCOAL

1. Bad breath: Charcoal is thought to cleanse the gastrointestinal tract that produces odors that are excreted through the lungs which cause bad breath.
2. Infections: Some individuals use charcoal to absorb bacteria, viruses, and toxins. They believe that it can act as a disinfectant in healing wounds.
3. Indigestion and Gas: It is thought to help relieve these problems when chewed or crushed and added to water.
4. Liver Congestion: Charcoal is thought by some to help eliminate the overload of toxins that the liver cannot filter.

Iridology

DIAGNOSIS WITH IRIDOLOGY

Iridology is not a method of treatment but rather of diagnosis. Iridology is the study of the iris of the eye to determine weaknesses in the body. Iridologists feel that areas of the iris correspond with different body parts. The iris of the eye is used as an indicator of the health of the body. Iridologists look for clarity, color, texture, fibers, rings and spots on the iris. The right and left irises are both used because they are thought to correspond to the right and left organs in the body.

HISTORY

This practice is thought to date back to the twelfth century when shepherds studied the eyes of sheep to determine the weak ones. Dr. Von Peczely is credited with making the first iridology chart in 1866. He did much research and studying before making detailed charts to determine the location of the problem in the body. Many others took part in establishing the field and practice of iridology. Other evidence has been found concerning the historical use of the study of the eye to determine the condition of the body. Medicine men in ancient America were known to spend time with individuals looking at the eye before giving a recommendation or remedy. Hippocrates noticed changes in the eye as changes in the body occurred and he promoted the use of herbs and natural methods to cure the body.

Iridologists feel that as the body begins to deteriorate, the iris perceives where and what is involved. This deterioration is reflected by a change in the iris. They believe that the eyes are the window to the body and all illness is accompanied by a change in the iris of the eye. Their theory is that serious problems surface in the iris before symptoms may become apparent. This allows the problem to be treated naturally before it becomes a serious condition.

This iris of the eye is thought to correspond to both internal and external areas of the body. By examining the specific areas of the iris, iridologists believe they can spot and identify different ailments in the body. The iris of the eye is full of nerve fibers which are connected to the brain. And the brain is in contact with the body parts through the flow of impulses through the nervous system.

Layers of the Eye

The iris of the eye has four different layers. Three of these are used and considered to be important in analyzing the condition of the body. They are: the anterior border layer, the stromal layer and the posterior eplithelium layer. The iridologist looks for pigment and pattern changes in the iris of the eye to determine a weakness. And different levels of change correspond to different types of problems.

Iridologists feel that the signs of weaknesses that appear in the iris of the eye indicate inherited conditions. They may not become visible until a child is five or six years old. Illnesses seem to arise out of those areas of weakness which are identified in the iris. Whether a particular weakness is manifest is dependent upon how the body is maintained. Iridologists feel that by eating a diet full of natural foods and using natural means of healing, the areas of weakness can be strengthened and corresponding illness avoided.

Most iridologists believe in the natural approach to healing. They feel that by using drugs, the body will build up toxins that can cause more serious problems. Iridologists believe in using effective but natural means to fill and fortify the body's needs. They pursue and advocate the use of herbs and changes in diet to achieve a healthy condition in the body. They feel that these natural substances have the necessary nutrients i.e.; vitamins, minerals, enzymes, and other substances, which are needed in the body to regain strength and health.

Diet and Nutrition

NUTRITION BASICS

THE THEORY OF CORRECT DIET

It is impossible to prescribe a correct diet which will work for everyone. And there are certainly contradictory theories concerning all types of nutritional regiments. Diets and nutritional information abound. Some claim a high protein diet is the answer. Others swear by a high fiber low carbohydrate routine. And some recommend high amounts of complex carbohydrates. But it is important to use common sense. Consider your own individual body needs. What is right for you now, may not work for your body in a few years. At different times in our lives, we need different amounts of specific nutrients.

Proper nutrition is an important contributing factor in the total health of the body. And it is necessary to pay attention to what is actually being consumed. This is one area in which we have control. We can make our dietary habits work for or against us.

Nutrients are divided into three basic categories. They include fats, carbohydrates, and protein.

Fats

Fats are the most calorie dense nutrient. They are made of carbon, hydrogen, and oxygen. Fats contain nine calories per gram. This is almost twice that found in carbohydrates and protein.

Body needs Fats

The human body needs fat in the diet to survive. But the amount needed is very small in relation to the overall diet. Many people enjoy foods high in fat. With the pace of life most of us live, we often choose to eat fast food which is usually high in fat. This life style full of high fat foods is not good for the body. High fat diets are responsible for contributing to many illnesses and disorders including some types of cancer, cardiovascular disease, intestinal problems, hypertension, and autoimmune diseases.

Uses of Fats

A small amount of fat is essential to a healthy body. A layer of fat insulates the body from the environment. Fat-soluble vitamins, A, D, E, and K, need dietary fat to be utilized by the body. Linoleic acid found in polyunsaturated fats such as grains, nuts, seeds, and some vegetables help the body metabolize fats. Fats are needed by the body cells to help perform many vital roles including brain function, the production of certain hormones, nerve impulses, and metabolism. And some forms of dietary fat such as linoleic acid, eicosapentaenoic acid, and linolenic acid all contribute to vital functions. Fats are important to the body; however, excess fat in the diet is detrimental to health. But the amount needed is small and can be obtained from eating a well balanced diet full of whole foods.

Types of Fats

Most of dietary fat falls under one of three categories of fatty acids: saturated, polyunsaturated, and monounsaturated. Most animal fat is composed of saturated fats. And most vegetable, seed, and nut oils consist of polyunsaturated and monounsaturated fatty acids.

Saturated Fats

Saturated fats are considered to be the least healthy for the body. Their composition causes them to become hard when refrigerated. The major contributor to saturated fats is animal fat. But some vegetable oils such as coconut and palm oils, are also high in saturated fat. Evidence is clear that a diet high in saturated fats can lead to many health problems. In cultures where there is little availability of saturated fats in the diet, there are few cases of coronary heart disease. In our American culture, the consumption of saturated fats is high. And we certainly see the results in the high number of individuals suffering from heart disease and atherosclerosis. A diet low in saturated fats is encouraged.

Polyunsaturated Fats

Polyunsaturated fats are usually recommended over saturated. But they also can cause problems. A theory known as the free radical theory states that certain areas of unsaturation in the chain of fatty acids are very vulnerable to attack by oxygen when exposed to the air, especially when heated. And this can release free radicals and peroxides. The free radicals are responsible for changing more of the fats to peroxides and the peroxides cause the production of more free radicals. These free radicals are very destructive and can cause damage to DNA and lead to cancer and premature aging. Polyunsaturated fats when used rather than saturated fats, are known to help lower cholesterol levels. But butter is thought to cause less damage because of its lower amounts of free radicals released when heated. So what is the answer? Probably a lower intake of all types of fats and choosing to use monounsaturated oils in small amounts.

MONOUNSATURATED FATS

Monounsaturated fats are considered by many to be the best to use in moderation. These include olive oil and canola oil. Considerable studies have been done using olive oil. It seems that olive oil is beneficial in lowering LDL cholesterol levels and not in lowering the HDL cholesterol levels which are beneficial and protective. Olive oils which are not refined are usually recommended because of their protection against oxidation and the release of free radicals.

LOW OVERALL FAT

A diet low in overall fat consumption is highly recommended. And using monunsaturated oils whenever possible in moderation. Small amounts of other fats may be consumed on a limited basis. The diet should not consist of more than 20 to 30 % of the calories in the form of fat. The ideal to shoot for is probably in the 10 to 15 % range. Remember to read the labels of products to learn the fat content.

Cholesterol

Cholesterol is a term that we are all familiar with. It brings fear into the minds of many. It is a waxlike substance which can accumulate in the arteries adhering to the arterial walls often near the heart. There are actually two types of cholesterol; low-density lipoproteins, or LDL, which is considered the bad cholesterol, and high-density lipoproteins, or HDL, which is thought to be the good cholesterol.

LDL CHOLESTEROL

LDL cholesterol is the type that can cause damage to the artery walls. It contains a chemical known as apolipoprotein B which is responsible for the problems. The LDL cholesterol along with the apolipoprotein B can adhere to the arterial walls causing plaque build up and allowing less blood to flow smoothly. When the adherence is near the heart, the individual is at risk of developing coronary heart disease.

HDL CHOLESTEROL

HDL cholesterol is thought to be the good cholesterol. It is considered to be beneficial in protecting the arteries. It may actually protect the cholesterol from adhering to the arterial walls. A high HDL level is helpful in preventing heart disease.

CHOLESTEROL FACTORS

Cholesterol is a substance which circulates through the body. It is controlled by the liver which can aid in removing the cholesterol from the blood and returning it to bile which aids in digestion. In the bile, the cholesterol can again be absorbed back into the bloodstream. The total cholesterol count is important because of the ratio between the HDL and the LDL.

Cholesterol count is affected by different circumstances. Heredity is thought to play a major role in cholesterol levels. Diet is also important. Most people who eat diets high in fat and cholesterol will have problems. There are a few who can get away with it due to highly efficient liver function. But most individuals should watch their cholesterol intake in order to lower the risk of heart disease. And following the basic nutritional guidelines by following a diet rich in vegetables, fruit, and whole grains will aid in controlling cholesterol levels. Exercise and stress management are also effective tools in lowering overall cholesterol levels in the blood.

Most individuals can lower the cholesterol levels by making changes in their life style such as diet, exercise and stress management. But some may require drug therapy to see a major change.

Carbohydrates

Carbohydrates in the past were thought to be largely responsible for problems with obesity. Experts recommended limiting all carbohydrates and starchy food to lose weight. But times have changed and this basic food group is known to be essential to health and weight loss.

SUGAR

The sugar in the carbohydrates are used for energy. All carbohydrates consist of one or more simple sugar combination. One is called a monosaccharide. When two combine, it is known as a disaccharide. And a combination of more than two simple sugars is called a polysaccharide. The polysaccharides are also known as complex carbohydrates.

SIMPLE CARBOHYDRATES

Simple carbohydrates are found in the form of different sugars including glucose, fructose, sucrose, and lactose. Complex carbohydrates are essential to health. They consist of whole grain products, rice, potatoes, pasta, corn, etc. These complex carbohydrates are important to the body and are a valuable source of energy.

COMPLEX CARBOHYDRATES

Complex carbohydrates are commonly known as starches. They are easily utilized as energy for the body. They are usually low in calories. Its the added fat and sugar that cause problems. For an active person the diet should consist of approximatley 50% in the form of complex carbohydrates.

When the carbohydrates are refined such as white flour and rice, they lose some of their value. They can still be valued as a source of energy but fiber and valuable nutrients are lost in the processing. It is important to include whole grain products to ensure a healthy diet.

SIMPLE SUGARS

Simple sugars are burned immediately by the body. This can cause large fluctuations in the blood sugar levels when large amounts are consumed. Insulin is required to remove the glucose from the blood. And this results in a sharp lowering of the blood sugar levels. The starches or complex carbohydrates take longer to digest and do not cause the same fluctuations. The body can store the starches and use the calories as needed.

Some forms of sugar considered natural, such as fructose, maple sugar, date sugar, honey and raw brown sugar, still cause blood sugar level fluctuations. Some may contain small amounts of vitamins and minerals, but they should still be used in moderation.

Proteins

Protein is found abundantly in the body. It has many important contributions to functions in the body. Protein helps with the growth and repair of tissue in the body including muscle and bone. They also help make up the complex cell structure.

AMINO ACIDS

Protein is broken down through the digestion process into amino acids. There are many different combinations of amino acids in the body. 22 of these are considered important for life. Eight of these cannot be manufactured from other amino acids and are considered essential amino acids. They must come from the diet on a daily basis.

PROTEIN NEEDS

Only a small amount of protein is needed in the diet. Most individuals get much more than the four ounces a day needed to sustain life. The excess is burned as energy. But protein is not considered to be an efficient source of energy. Protein involves a complex combination of molecules. It takes longer for the body to digest and use this energy. High amounts of protein in the body put extra stress and work on the digestive system contributing to feelings of fatigue. Protein contains nitrogen which must be eliminated from the body through the work of the liver and kidneys. This is stressful on those organs of the body.

PROTEIN SOURCES

Proteins in the form of legumes, vegetables, and grains do not contain all the essential amino acids. But by combining incomplete proteins, all the essential amino acids can be consumed.

Protein should be eaten in moderation from meat sources especially those high in saturated fat such as red meat. Poultry contains less fat especially when the excess fat and skin are removed. Fish is a good source of protein but be careful of contamination. Eggs are high in protein but the yolks do contain cholesterol. They should not be eaten on a daily basis. Legumes which include peas, beans, lentils, and soy products, are good sources of protein.

Whole grain products contain some protein. They can be eaten with other protein foods. Nuts and seeds are high in protein but also contain high amounts of fat.

COMBINATIONS

Complete proteins in a given day can be supplied by these combinations: corn and beans; rice and beans; grains and legumes; grains and seeds; or seeds and legumes. Of course, varying amounts of amino acids are found in most natural foods. Avoiding junk food and concentrating on nutritious foods can ensure the body's efficient utilization of protein.

COMPLEMENTARY PROTEINS

If complementary proteins are eaten throughout the day, the body can assimilate them and extract the amino acids it needs to regenerate the daily requirements needed. Protein from plant sources can be more easily assimilated than the protein found in meats. Protein requirements can be met if a wide variety of vegetables, grain, legumes, fruits, and a little meat are consumed.

The synthetic hormones found in animal products such as milk, cheese, eggs, and meat can cause problems. Excessive estrogen from these sources, when not eliminated by the liver can lead to breast cancer, as well as cancer of the reproductive system and many other problems. Too much protein from animal sources may cause problems such as constipation, autotoxemia, hyperactivity, nutritional deficiencies, kidney damage, heart disease, and cancer.

The most important information to remember is to eat a nutritionally balanced diet including ample amounts of complex carbohydrates, some protein, and just a little fat.

Enzymes

CATALYSTS

Enzymes are the protein-like substances formed in plants and animals. They act as catalysts in chemical reactions. Enzymes speed up the processes in the body.

Glands and organs in the body depend on the activity of the enzymes to function properly Enzymes are found in all living things. There are around 700 different enzymes which function in the body. They each perform a different function. Enzymes are found in the food we eat and supply energy for the body. Enzymes are found in raw, live food. This includes fresh fruits and vegetables. When the valuable enzymes are missing in the body, the glands must try and manufacture the ones it needs. This can cause the glands to over work and cause feelings of fatigue and exhaustion.

There are four main categories of food enzymes. These include:

1. Lipase (which serves to break down fat)
2. Protease (which breaks down protein)
3. Cellulase (which assists in breaking down cellulose)
4. Amylase (which breaks down starch)

Amino Acids

BUILDING BLOCKS

Amino acids are considered the building blocks of protein. Proteins are substances which occur in all living matter. A proper balance of amino acids can benefit the blood, skin, immune system, and digestive system. Amino acids can also help with neurotransmitters in the brain, helping to stabilize moods and balance transmissions in the brain.

There are eight essential amino acids and twenty-four complementary ones which work synergistically to promote health in the body. Carnitine is an example of an amino acid which helps to metabolize fat and reduce triglycerides. Carnitine is synthesized from the combination of the amino acids lysine and methionine.

Methionine helps remove heavy metals from the tissue. Lead is one heavy metal which causes brain damage.

Fiber

Fiber has come to the public's attention through medical advice and the media. It is certainly an important item that was neglected for a period of time and considered non essential. Fiber has always been considered important in the natural nutritional world. Processed foods were introduced, and we were all hooked. But now more attention is being placed on fiber and its importance. And this is one area in which the medical community and natural health field agree.

RECENT APPRECIATION OF FIBER

Fiber, for a period of time, was considered by modern medicine as non-essential in our diets. In fact, it was removed from foods to make them smooth and more appetizing. Fiber was thought to have no nutritional benefits. But times have changed and more and more people are realizing the healthy contribution fiber can make in their diets. This is another example of the balance required in our lives. A natural approach to health allows us to take advantage of natures wisdom even before modern medicine discovers why the natural approach works.

CELL WALLS OF PLANTS

Fiber consists of the cell walls of plants. Plants are supported by these that keep them rigid. Every plant cell has a wall of fibers. It is usually considered to be the parts of the foods we eat that are not digestible. This is the material that is important in keeping the digestive process moving and the intestinal system functioning efficiently.

INSOLUBLE FIBER

Fiber consists of both water-insoluble fibers which absorb water swelling and adding bulk. Some of these include celluloses, ligning, and hemicelluloses found in whole grains and vegetables.

SOLUBLE FIBER

Water-soluble are found in apples, citrus fruits, oats, legumes, and some vegetables.They are known as gums, pectins, and mucilages.

Studies have been conducted making fantastic claims to the importance of fiber. Lower cholesterol levels have been attributed to fiber intake as well as the prevention of heart disease and colon cancer. The important thing to remember is that most people do not get enough fiber. The National Cancer Institute has recommended that people eat at least 20 to 35 grams of fiber each day. And many experts suggest as much as 40 grams per day. The average American probably only consumes around 10 to 15 grams of fiber per day.

HIGH FIBER DIETS

In cultures where fruits, vegetables, and whole grains are eaten in abundance, there is less incidence of obesity, colitis, cancer and polyps of the colon, and appendicitis. Experts attribute this to the high fiber content contained in the diets of these people. The fiber adds bulk and the elimination time is increased speeding up the process. It seems that the quicker the food is eliminated through the system, the greater the benefits. Fiber can keep the toxins from building up in the colon by keeping the bowels moving. High protein and fat diets are absorbed mainly in the intestines. This may lead to constipation problems. Also cholesterol and fats are excreted from the body at a faster pace as well as toxins. The theory is that the less time toxins and carcinogenic substances remain in the bowels, the less chance of them causing problems. Diets low in dietary fiber allow the food to remain longer in the intestines causing toxins to build up and maybe disease to begin. The fiber will not cure cancer, but it may help in preventing problems for susceptible individuals. With a high fiber diet, the bowel wall may remain strong and clean.

FIBER FOODS

The best method of increasing fiber is to include whole grains, brown rice, oats, pasta, and ample amounts of fruits and vegetables to the diet. Be aware of what you are eating. Fast foods are not only high in fat, but very low in fiber. Fiber should be gradually introduced into the diet as to avoid intestinal problems such as diarrhea, bloating, and flatulence.

OAT BRAN

Dr. James W. Anderson M.D. a professor at the University of Kentucky College of Medicine is credited with his research on high fiber diets with diabetics. He noticed that oat bran was bringing down their insulin requirements as well as their blood cholesterol levels.

The dose of oat bran was very high. He used a diet of 100 g. of oat bran a day which is about one cup of dry oat bran. Blood cholesterol levels dropped about 20% in this study. The patients also lost weight. Practically, this is a much cheaper and healthier way to lower blood cholesterol.

APPENDICITIS

Patricia Hausman and Judith Benn Hurley in their book THE HEALING FOODS published by Rodale Press, at pages 35-36, suggest how fiber can prevent appendicitis:

"Of all possible dietary explanations for appendicitis, a low fiber intake has been suspected most. The case for a protective effect from fiber rests on facts such as these. Appendicitis tends to be more common in countries where the diet is low in fiber. During the war, when appendicitis rates fell, residents of Switzerland and the English Channel Islands were eating more fiber (and less fat) than usual. Surveys in African cities by Denis Burkitt, M.D., have shown that appendicitis is ten times more common in whites than in blacks. In Africa, of course, the former are more likely to follow a Western-type diet. Some research shows that children who develop appendicitis eat less fiber. Jean Brender, Ph.D., and associates at the University of Washington School of Public Health reported in 1985 that children who had eaten the diets richest in fiber were only half as likely to develop the disease."

Diabetes

Diabetic control is often made easier if the person is put on a high fiber diet. Eating foods rich in soluble fiber slows the absorption of food in the blood stream. This helps stop the swing in blood sugar levels.

Constipation

Adding fiber to the diet will often end constipation problems. Insoluble fiber will add bulk and start intestinal movement. Constipation can be the cause of toxin build-up and disease. So fiber can help keep the colon functioning.

Colon Cancer

Research has shown that low fiber diets can cause food residue to become hard and remain in the colon for long periods of time. If this mass contains some carcinogenic material, it could make contact with the bowel. When a person eats plenty of fiber, the colon flows more uniformly and the food digestion is more rapid. It is sensible to eat a high fiber diet which is low in fat content. The two combined can help reduce the risk of colon cancer. Though nothing is certain, common sense will tell us to eat nutritional food high in fiber which are also often low in fat.

HEMORRHOIDS

This problem seems to be associated with a low fiber diet. Constipation and straining appear to lead to this problem. The pressure from straining can cause the veins in the anal area to swell and this is known as hemorrhoids. So a high fiber diet along with exercise can do wonders for this problem.

OBESITY

Individuals put on high fiber, low fat diets generally lose weight at a slow and healthy rate. People on a high fiber, unrefined diet absorb less of the energy they take in the form of food. Fiber increases the amount of energy and fat passed in the stools. They may also prevent the complete absorption of food because the fiber foods pass through the bowel more quickly. Researchers are finding that obesity is not so much a problem of how much we eat but of what we eat.

Salt

FOOD ADDITIVE

Salt is considered to be one of the leading food additives. Most people love the taste of salty foods. Sodium chloride is the official name of common table salt. The actual requirement of salt in the body is approximately one quarter teaspoon per day. But most people in the United States consume much more than that. The amount is estimated to be about 20 times that which is needed. The body does require salt but only in small amounts. And excessive quantities are associated with many disorders in the body including hypertension, depression, edema, obesity, headaches, and kidney problems.

SODIUM

Sodium is the negative factor in salt. It is required in small amounts by the body to help with the conduction of nerve impulses, fluid regulation in the body, and the heart.

Patients suffering from hypertension and heart problems are often put on salt restricted diets. The medical community has declared a war on excessive salt and encourages use only in moderation and for some, not at all. Low sodium products are on the market. And many health conscious individuals are looking for ways to control their salt intake.

The best advice is to eat less processed food. Restaurant food is also known for high salt content. Salt is often added in high amounts. And try not to add salt to foods cooked at home. There is enough salt found naturally in foods to fill the needs of the body. The salt habit can be kicked gradually. In moderation it is usually acceptable for most individuals.

Sugar

There are many forms of sugar both raw and refined. Food must taste good to sell, and so sugar has become a popular additive to many commercial foods. Sugar is an easy way to make food taste good. All forms of sugar belong to the carbohydrate family. They all have similar molecular structures which include a carbon atom attached to hydrogen and oxygen.

GLUCOSE

The body makes glucose by breaking down carbohydrate foods. These include fruits, vegetables, and grains. Carbohydrates are the greatest source of energy for the body. They are necessary for the process of digestion and the assimilation of nutrients taken into the body.

Digestion changes carbohydrates into glucose. This glucose goes to the pancreas where the increase in the blood glucose level stimulates the production of insulin. The insulin is carried by the bloodstream to the liver where the excess glucose is converted to glycogen which is stored in the liver until the liver is full to capacity.

Insulin/Diabetis

If the insulin supply by the pancreas is too great, too much glucose will be converted to glycogen. The blood glucose level will remain low. This is known as hypoglycemia. This is caused by eating too many simple sugars.

When the pancreas supplies too little insulin, the liver cannot convert excess glucose to glycogen. This condition is diabetes. The pancreas wears out from producing insulin to neutralize sugar foods. Sugar builds up in the blood and the blood glucose level rises and remains high.

Sugar and Nutrients

Sugar robs the body of valuable nutrients. When sugar is eaten often and in excess, the body produces an acidic condition. In this acidic state more and more minerals are required to keep the body in balance. The body uses calcium from the bones which leaves the body (including the teeth) in a weakened condition. To metabolize refined sugar, the body finds the missing nutrients from other sources. These can be from foods eaten in the same meal or from the body tissue itself. We lose vitamins and minerals, especially vitamin B, calcium, phosphorous and iron from our own body reserve.

Sugar Addiction

Sugar is eaten in excess by many Americans. It is one of the most destructive elements in our diets. It acts as a drug and is very addictive. The more you eat the more you crave. These cravings can be satisfied with vegetables, fruits and grains. Some sweeteners seem to be absorbed slower and may cause less havoc in the body. Some sweeteners also contain nutrients and do not deplete the body of its own resources.

Sucrose

Sucrose is refined white sugar or common table sugar. It is made from sugar cane an sugar beets. When sugar cane and sugar beets are refined, the results is almost pure sucrose. Each sucrose molecule is made of one fructose molecule and one dextrose molecule. Americans consume about 100-140 pounds of this white sugar per year. Sucrose contains no protein, minerals or vitamins. It is almost 100% pure simple carbohydrate. It quickly turns to glucose in the body.

Raw Sugar

Raw sugar is brown in color. This color means that some nutrients remain. It is in a granular form. Raw sugar is obtained from the evaporation of sugar cane juice. This sugar is then refined and produces white sugar or sucrose.

Brown Sugar

Brown sugar is made of sugar crystals in a molasses syrup with natural flavor and color. Most of the brown sugar in the United States simply consists of white refined sugar with a little molasses added for color. A small amount of nutrients are added to the refined sugar through the molasses.

Corn Syrup

Corn syrup is produced by adding enzymes to cornstarch. High fructose corn syrup comes form corn. The amount of fructose in the corn syrup will vary between manufactures. And the rest of the corn syrup is dextrose. it is used as a sweetener often to prevent other sugars from forming crystals when they cool.

DEXTROSE

Dextrose is the same as glucose. It is made from synthetic starch by the action of heat and enzymes.

LACTOSE

Lactose is milk sugar. It occurs naturally in the milk of all mammals. It is made from whey.

FRUCTOSE

Fructose is also known as levulose. It is a commercially produced sugar which has the same molecular structure as fructose naturally found in fruit and honey. It is made from sucrose which is composed of fructose and glucose. So basically the glucose is taken out which leaves the fructose. Studies have supported the belief that fructose does not seem to stimulate insulin production by the pancreas. When fructose enters the bloodstream, it does not seem to require insulin to get into the cells. Some of the fructose is metabolized in the liver. Some portions of fructose are converted to glycogen which eventually is changed to glucose and does require insulin. But this is a much slower process and causes the glucose to enter the bloodstream at a slow and even rate. Fructose is thought by many to not cause the large fluctuations in blood glucose levels and causes less stress on the pancreas than sucrose.

MOLASSES

Blackstrap molasses is the syrup that remains after sugar is crystallized out of sugar cane juice. The process is repeated many times to get all the color and nutrients out. Molasses is the residue that contains the minerals and vitamins from sugar cane. Blackstrap molasses contains calcium, phosphorus, iron, sodium, potassium, thiamine, riboflavin, and niacin. It can be used as a sugar substitute.

HONEY

Honey is a complex sugar consisting mainly of fructose and glucose with some minerals and vitamins. It contains no protein or fat.

Honey varies in flavor depending on what flower nectar it is from. It contains different sugars from the nectar as well as additives from the bee's digestive system. These work as a preservative which allows honey to keep for a long period of time. Honey is absorbed slower than other sugars because of its high fructose content.

Studies have shown that bacteria cannot grow in honey because of its potassium content. This mineral absorbs the liquid in which the bacteria need to survive. It can be used to prevent infections. It is soothing to the skin tissue and has been used effectively as a treatment for burns.

Honey has been used as a folk remedy. It is a great tasting alternative to other sweeteners.

Maple Syrup

Maple syrup is found in three different grades. Grad A is mild tasting and sweet but contains less minerals. Grade B has more minerals and maple taste. Grade C is the highest in minerals but has a very strong maple taste.The vitamin and mineral content varies depending on where the syrup is from.

Some experts feel that there is no special advantage to eating any specific type of sugar. There are some differences, but they can all cause problems when used in extreme amounts. Remember to use moderation when using sugar in all forms. It is important to pay attention to your sugar intake no matter what form it is in. This includes fruit, fruit juices, ice cream, candy or prepared foods.

Artificial Sweeteners

There is a lot of controversy regarding the use of artificial sweeteners. Many support the belief that these sweeteners have many advantages over natural forms of sugar.

ASPARTAME

NutraSweet™ and *Equal*™ are the trade names for aspartame. Advocates claim that aspartame is natural made from two building blocks of protein similar to those found in fruits, vegetables, grains, and dairy products. But others claim that this product is far from natural. It is composed of two amino acids which are phenylalanine and aspartic acid and found in nature. But the problems seems to be that they are isolated from the other amino acids that they usually are found in combination with. And the two amino acids that aspartame does contain are delivered in the body in a highly concentrated form which the body does not ordinarily have to deal with.

SWEETER THAN SUGAR

Artificial sweeteners are hundreds of times sweeter than sugar. And some researchers believe that the body is tricked into thinking it is getting a large amount of sugar. This causes the metabolic process to speed up leaving the individual hungry and tired. And this in return may cause more food to be eaten. Some studies have shown that dieters who use artificial sweeteners may actually gain more weight than those eating regular sugar products.

In HEALTH AND FITNESS EXCELLENCE, published by Houghton Mifflin Company, 1989 on page 340, and written by Robert K. Cooper Ph.D, states, "Don't rely on artificially sweetened foods and beverages to help you lose weight or prevent fat gain. According to an ongoing study by the American Cancer Society involving more than 78,000 women aged fifty to sixty-nine, long-term users of artificial sweeteners are more likely to gain weight than nonusers over the course of one year. In addition, fake sweeteners usually don't satisfy hunger. A recent study on aspartame conducted at Leeds University in England reported that not only was this sweetener generally ineffective in suppressing appetite, but in some people it actually increased feelings of hunger. In contrast, sugar (glucose) was found to reduce hunger and produce a feeling of fullness."

Some information has brought to light some new facts about aspartame. It contains the amino acid phenylalanine. It is known to cause problems with some of the brain neurotransmitters. It seems to affect some of the brain levels of amino acids and affects the production and release of some neurotransmissions. This could affect many different brain functions such as blood pressure, appetite, and mood changes.

Side Affects

There are also some who have claimed other side affects associated with the use of aspartame. These include dizziness, nausea, diarrhea, headaches, seizures, and mood changes. Reports have been sent to the National Center for Disease Control concerning this issue. And the company responsible has also been sent many complaints.

Cyclamates

Cyclamates which were banned some years ago, but are now being reconsidered. Saccharin is know to cause cancer and is still present as an artificial sweetener.

Most natural health advocates recommend using natural sugar in small amounts and staying away from artificial sweeteners. There is really no evidence to support the use of artificial sweeteners as beneficial. And the studies done seem to show that more weight is gained by individuals who choose to use artificial sweeteners.

Variety in Diet

Eating a variety of foods will help the body get the nutrients that it needs and also make meal time more enjoyable. There are a wide variety of fruits and vegetables available in the supermarket which are nutritious and delicious. Fresh fruits and vegetables are full of nutrients. Canned, dried, and frozen foods often lose some of their nutritional value through the processing procedure. Additives also can be undesirable. Remember to wash thoroughly or peel produce that has been treated with pesticides.

Vegetables and Fruits

Vegetables and fruits are important to a balanced and nutritional diet. They are full of vitamins, minerals, enzymes, protein, complex carbohydrates, and fiber. There are many different varieties available.

If possible, it is important to buy produce that is free of pesticides. Or grow as much produce as possible to ensure quality and safety. Local farmers can be used to be sure of the freshness of the produce.

Try and introduce new types of produce to the family. There are many exotic and different varieties available at the local supermarket. Prepare them in an attractive manner.

Raw as well as cooked vegetables should be included in the diet. Some should be cooked to make sure that the natural toxins are eliminated. These include broccoli, collards, kale, and brussels sprouts. Carrots, onions, garlic, salad greens, cucumbers, radishes, peppers, and tomatoes are great eaten raw. Again, variety is the key. Vegetables are essential to a healthy body.

Fruits should be sun ripened if possible. Unfortunately they are usually picked green and allowed to ripen on the way to the grocery store. This does not allow for the optimum amount of nutrients. Using the local farmer makes it possible to acquire sun ripened fruit.

Whole Grains

More and more research and the medical community are pointing to the benefits of a diet rich in whole grain products. Processed foods are slowly losing their attractiveness in the eyes of many consumers. Whole wheat bread sales are on the rise. And there are a variety of delicious and nutritious grains available. It is now known that whole grains are important to ensure a nutritionally sound diet.

Complex Carbohydrates

Grains are known to be low in fat and rich in complex carbohydrates. They have been used by many people in many cultures as a staple in the diet. They can be used to make all kinds of wonderful recipes. And they are a low cost source of nutrition, fiber, vitamins, and minerals.

They are best when grown organically to avoid contamination and pesticides. Grains can be cooked, sprouted, and ground into flour for making baked goods.

Whole Wheat

Whole wheat is probably the best known grain in our culture. It is full of nutritional value. It is often used for baking bread. Some use wheat in recipes as a meat substitute. And whole wheat can be used in soups and as a cereal. Most people are accustomed to the white flour which is the processed form of whole wheat. Unfortunately, the fiber and germ are eliminated in the processing. The whole grain wheat is a valuable nutrient.

MILLET

Millet is a grain that has been used in many cultures. It is the only grain that is considered to be a complete protein. It can be added to cereals and breads and combined with other grains.

BROWN RICE

Brown rice is a nutritious addition to the diet. Brown rice needs to cook longer than white rice but the wait is worth the time. Most people are used to the white rice commonly used. But brown rice can be introduced and enjoyed by most everyone. It is full of nutritional value.

BUCKWHEAT

Buckwheat is a valuable grain. It is used as the main grain product in many northern European countries. The seeds of the buckwheat flower are ground in to flour to make cereal and pancakes. Buckwheat is a hardy grain and it thrives in adverse conditions. It has few problems with insects and diseases and seems to do well even in poor soil.

BARLEY

Barley is a wonderful and nutritious addition to soups and stews. It is a member of the same family as corn, oats, rice, and wheat. Barley flour is used in bread, cereal and as a thickening agent.

CORN

Corn is the only vegetable that is also considered a grain. Ground corn is great for muffins, tortillas, cereal and breads. It is also used as livestock feed and to make nonfood items such as drugs, paints, and paper goods. There are several thousand different types and varieties of corn.

OATS

Oats are a very important grain. The seeds of the plant are used in oatmeal, cookies, breads, and cereals. Oats have a high food value. The majority of the crop grown in the United States is fed to livestock. But oats are becoming more popular with the interest in the health benefits of whole grain oats and oat bran.

Rye

Rye is similar to wheat. Rye is used to make delicious breads. It is thought to have been cultivated from wild species found in Asia. Rye does not contain as much gluten as wheat and is preferred by some for this reason.

Legumes, Nuts, and Seeds

Legumes include peas, beans, and lentils. They are an inexpensive and nutritious addition to the diet. They contain complex carbohydrates, fiber, protein, vitamins, and minerals. They are low in fat and cholesterol.

Nuts and seeds are recommended only in small amounts because of their high content of fat. They are a good source of protein and fiber and contain some essential fatty acids, vitamins, and minerals.

VITAMINS AND MINERALS

The Importance of Vitamins

Vitamins are complex organic substances needed by the body, often in small amounts, for good health. They are in fact necessary for life. Vitamins work with the body to perform life giving functions. Vitamins work as coenzymes activating the process which take place continually in the body. Vitamins are essential parts of the enzymes which make things happen in the body. Deficiencies of vitamins must be corrected because of the important functions they perform in the body process.

DEFICIENCY FACTORS

Different factors can contribute to vitamin and mineral deficiencies. Some include air pollution, pain, stress, drug therapy, illness, and a nutritional deficient diet. So it is important to be aware of deficiencies that may occur and correct them.

Vitamin and mineral therapy is natural. It involves using substances the body needs to function and heal. They help to put the body in a position to heal and maintain.

The medical community is becoming aware of the healing power of vitamins. In the April 6, 1992 issue of TIME magazine the cover article contained information on vitamins. Janice M. Horowitz, Elaine Lafferty, and Dick Thompson combined their efforts in this excellent article. They state, "Most of the excitement, however, is being generated by a group of vitamins — C, E, and beta carotene, the chemical parent of Vitamin A— that are known as antioxidants. These nutrients appear to be able to defuse the volatile toxic molecules, known as oxygen-free radicals, that are a byproduct of normal metabolism in cells. These molecules are also created in the body by exposure to sunlight, x-rays, ozone, tobacco smoke, car exhaust and other environmental pollutants.

Free radicals are cellular renegades; they wreck havoc by damaging DNA, altering biochemical compounds, corroding cell membranes and killing cells outright. Such molecular mayhem, scientists increasingly believe, plays a major role in the development of ailments like cancer, heart or lung disease and cataracts. Many researchers are convinced that the cumulative effects of free radicals also underline the gradual deterioration that is the hallmark of aging in all individuals, healthy as well as sick. Antioxidants, studies suggest, might help stem the damage by neutralizing free radicals. In effect they perform as cellular sheriffs, collaring the radicals and hauling them away."

VITAMINS IN DIET

Vitamins must be obtained from out diets. They are contained in the food we eat, herbs and supplements. Vitamins are used in the body constantly and must be replaced daily.

Vitamins help the body use other nutrients. They contribute to the breaking down of protein, carbohydrates and fats into usable forms. The body must have a balance of vitamins to function properly.

WATER/FAT SOLUBLE

Vitamins are either water or fat soluble. Most fall into the water soluble category. This means they combine with water in the body to function and then are excreted in the urine. Water soluble vitamins are used by the body immediately. They are quickly excreted from the body.These vitamins only remain in the system for two to three hours and must be taken regularly whether in the food we eat or as a supplement.

Vitamins A,D, E, F and K are considered fat soluble. They remain in the body for a longer period of time. They combine with fats to be absorbed in the body. They are often stored in fat tissue in the body. Toxicity can occur if these fat soluble vitamins are taken in large doses for long periods of time. But cases of toxicity are extremely rare.

Vitamins should be taken before meals for proper absorption in the body. Vitamins work together in the body and should be combined for the most benefit.

VITAMIN COMBINATIONS

Jack Ritchason in his book THE VITAMIN AND HEALTH ENCYCLOPEDIA published by Woodland Books, 1986 on page 30, gives some examples of effective vitamin combinations.

"Vitamin A functions best with B-complex, vitamin D, vitamin E, calcium, phosphorus, and zinc.

Vitamin D functions best with vitamin A, vitamin C, choline, calcium, and phosphorus.

Vitamin E functions best with B-complex, inositol, vitamin C, manganese and selenium.

Vitamin C functions best with bioflavonoids, calcium, and magnesium.

Folic Acid functions best with B-complex and vitamin C.

Niacin functions best with vitamin B_1, vitamin B_2, B-complex and vitamin C.

Vitamin B_1 functions best with B-complex, vitamin B_2, folic acid, niacin, vitamin C and vitamin E.

Vitamin B_2 functions best with vitamin B_6, B-complex, vitamin C, and niacin.

Vitamin B_6 functions best with vitamin B_1, vitamin B_2, B-complex, pantothenic acid, vitamin C, and magnesium.

Vitamin B_{12} functions best with vitamin B_6, B-complex, vitamin C, folic acid, choline, inositol, and potassium.

Calcium functions best with vitamin A, vitamin C, vitamin D, iron, magnesium, and phosphorus.

Phosphorus functions best with calcium, vitamin A, vitamin D, iron, and manganese.

Iron functions best with vitamin B_{12}, folic acid, vitamin C, and calcium.

Magnesium functions best with vitamin B_6, vitamin C, vitamin D, calcium and phosphorus.

Zinc functions best with vitamin A, calcium, and phosphorus."

The following list some information and benefits of essential vitamins.

VITAMIN A

Vitamin A is fat soluble which means it requires fats to be absorbed properly. It can be stored by the body but in extremely high doses taken over a prolonged period of time can be toxic.

Vitamin A is considered to be a yellow solid that makes up a portion of the cell membranes. It is contained in the thin lipid-protein material that surrounds each cell in the body. This essential vitamin is important in the protection process and monitoring what is allowed into each cell.

It helps maintain and repair healthy tissue, fight infection, counteracts night blindness, treat skin problems, and aids in the growth and maintenance of healthy bones, skin, teeth, and gums. It is thought to be an important factor in the formation of epithelial tissue. This tissue is found in the skin, glands, mucous membranes, respiratory tract, digestive tract and reproductive organs.

IMMUNE SYSTEM

Another important function of vitamin A is thought to be its ability to strengthen the immune system. It is known to improve resistance to infection and also to shorten the duration of infections that attack the body. When the body is attacked by an illness, the level of vitamin A in the body is deficient. This leaves the body vulnerable to a more severe reaction or infection. Many take vitamin A regularly to boost the immune system.

Vitamin A is also being recognized as a cancer preventive. It has been shown that vitamin A was effective in lowering the incidence of lung cancer among a group of male smokers. It may also decrease the development and spread of many different types of cancer.

EYE-SIGHT

Vitamin A has many important functions in the body. It is well known for its ability to counteract night blindness and healing other vision and eye problems. It helps maintain a substance known as visual purple in the eye which is needed to see in the dark. It may stop the progression of macular degeneration which is a common cause of blindness in older individuals.

SKIN HEALTH

Vitamin A has been used by dermatologists in treating skin disorders such as acne, psoriasis, and boils. It can be taken internally or applied directly to the problem area. It is known to maintain and repair healthy tissue. The skin needs vitamin A to keep it smooth, healthy, and moist. Dry and wrinkled skin can benefit from vitamin A by retarding the effects of exposure and aging.

HEALING

Vitamin A is thought to help in the healing process of bones and organs when damage has been done. It may also help in the growth and repair of healthy bones, hair, teeth, and gums.

BETA CAROTENE

Beta carotene is converted into vitamin A in the body. The carotene is the pigment which gives vegetables and fruits their yellow coloring. Beta carotene is also found in green vegetables but their coloring is from the chlorophyll. Some of the fruits and vegetables contain carotenes that are more easily used by the body. They each have a different level of utilization efficiency. Beta carotene seems to be most easily converted to vitamin A and thus, more efficiently used by the body. Beta carotene is a water soluble form of vitamin A. The body has the ability to use the Beta carotene as needed. And some believe that Beta carotene can be more effective than vitamin A alone in protecting against diseases such as cancer. There is evidence to support this theory. And many now believe that Beta carotene when converted to vitamin A in the body can help reduce the risk of breast, lung, colon, prostate, and cervical cancer. It may also benefit and prevent heart disease and strokes.

Vitamin A is found in fish liver oil, liver, green and yellow vegetables, eggs, milk, carrots, apricots, and sweet potatoes.

B-COMPLEX VITAMINS

The B-complex vitamins consist of B_1 (thiamin), B_2 (riboflavin), B_3(Niacin and niacinamide), B_5 (pantothenic acid), B_6 (pyridoxine), B_{12} (cobalamin), folic acid, biotin, choline, inositol, and PABA. Each of the B-complex vitamins work individually but they have similar roles and properties. They work together in the body and are often found in the same foods. These are needed in plentiful supply to ensure health and energy that the body needs. The B vitamins are essential to the nervous system and the emotional stability of individuals. These are water soluble vitamins.

VITAMIN B_1 (THIAMINE)

Vitamin B_1 is water soluble and needed by the body in only small amounts on a daily basis. It is often called the "Morale" vitamin because of its effect on mental health. People suffering from mental illness such as depression, paranoia, and confusion have responded positively to thiamine therapy. It is known for its ability to help strengthen the nervous system.

It helps the body metabolize carbohydrates. A diet high in carbohydrates whether complex or simple needs an increase in thiamine. This vitamin is needed to help assimilate the carbohydrates.

It is also thought to help increase the appetite and aid in the digestive process.

Vitamin B_1 has been used successfully in treating individuals suffering from alcoholism and drug addiction. It is also thought to help build the immune system and increase resistance to infection.

It is found in organ meats, dried beans, brown rice, whole grains, peas, whole wheat, oatmeal, peanuts, sunflower seeds, rice bran, wheat germ, millet, brewer's yeast, and blackstrap molasses.

VITAMIN B_2 (RIBOFLAVIN)

Vitamin B_2 helps the body digest and assimilate fats, proteins, and carbohydrates. It aids in metabolizing protein by helping to form enzymes which are needed in order to take oxygen to the cells.

It is essential for proper bone and tissue growth. Vitamin B_2 is involved in repairing tissue after an injury or illness causing damage. Some of these situations include burns, wounds, surgery, tuberculosis, fever, and malignancies.

Vitamin B_2 is considered to help with the potassium and sodium balance in the blood. It is also involved in the body's ability to absorb iron. And it could help in this case in preventing or correcting cases of anemia involving iron deficiencies.

Vitamin B_2 is helpful in maintaining good vision and in alleviating eye fatigue. It is found in the pigment of the retina and is involved in the eyes adjusting to light. A deficiency may lead to eye problems and even cataracts.

It is useful in promoting healthy growth of hair, skin, and nails. Dandruff may be a sign of vitamin B_2 deficiency. And an increase in B_2 along with the other B-vitamins have helped some overcome their dandruff problems.

It is found in almonds, dairy products, dry

hot red peppers, wheat germ, wild rice, eggs, meat, spinach, dried peas, liver, fish, white beans, millet, parsley, and sesame seeds.

VITAMIN B_3 (NIACINAMIDE OR NIACIN)

Vitamin B_3 is known to help promote healthy nerve function and brain function. A lack of vitamin B_3 may lead to mental problems or personality changes. This vitamin has been used to treat schizophrenia and autism in children with some success. There are some psychiatric doctors who use supplements including Niacin along with drugs in treating mental disorders. It may also help to increase memory and improve mental function involving senility.

Vitamin B_3 is an important element of the hormonal system. It aids the body in producing cortisone, thyroxine, insulin, and male and female sex hormones.

Niacin is thought to help regulate blood levels. This can help in the prevention of high cholesterol, high blood pressure, arteriosclerosis, and heart disease. It can help improve blood circulation. A number of studies indicate the effectiveness of Vitamin B_3 in reducing cholesterol and triglyceride levels in the blood. And some health practitioners are now choosing to use this vitamin to treat patients with cholesterol problems rather than using the traditional medications which are expensive and can cause side effects.

Some forms of niacin are not easily absorbed by the body. The body can usually produce enough of this vitamin on its own if enough vitamins B_1, B_2, and B_6 are available. But it must be replaced daily in the body.

Rice and wheat bran, dairy products, sesame seeds, sunflower seeds, liver, kidney, fish, eggs, potatoes, broccoli, tomatoes, carrots, white meat, avocados, whole wheat, and prunes all contain vitamin B_3.

VITAMIN B_5 (PANTOTHENIC ACID)

Vitamin B_5 is generally known as pantothenic acid. It is important in the production of hormones and the health of the adrenal gland. It is thought to be a factor in stimulating the pituitary gland in producing a natural form of cortisone.

"Panto" means everywhere and pantothenic acid is found in every living cell in the body. It is known to aid in the production of new cell growth and in maintaining normal growth and a regulator of growth stimulation.

Along with other vitamins, pantothenic acid is known to help in the metabolism of fats, carbohydrates, and proteins. It is essential to the digestion process and in converting foods into usable forms of energy.

Pantothenic acid is considered to be a contributor in fighting infection and disease and in speeding recovery after an illness or injury. It may also help the body hold up during injury or surgery.

This vitamin is also thought to help with resistance to stress and fatigue. This may be due in part to the connection with the adrenal gland and hormone production. It may be due to the nerve transmission involvement of pantothenic acid.

Some foods which contain this vitamin are brewer's yeast, molasses, egg yolks, soybeans, peanuts, wheat germ, whole grains, salt water fish, pork, beef, chicken, green vegetables, tomatoes, and potatoes.

VITAMIN B_6 (PYRODIXINE HYDROCHLORIDE)

Vitamin B_6 is an essential vitamin. It is involved in many enzyme functions and in the metabolism of amino acids. It is thought to be important in converting protein foods into amino acids. It is used in almost all body functions.

Vitamin B_6 is necessary for the production of red blood cells and antibodies. It aids the body in converting iron into hemoglobin in the blood. It is generally known to promote healthy blood and vessels.

As with other B vitamins, B_6 is essential to the function of the nervous system. It is necessary for the production of serotonin and neurotransmitters in the brain which are needed for proper brain function.

Foods which contain this essential vitamin include fish, peas, meat, chicken, avocado, cantaloupe, whole grains, brewer's yeast, wheat germ, blackstrap molasses, honey, liver, egg yolks, almonds, carrots, spinach, liver, millet, bananas, and leafy green vegetables.

VITAMIN B_9 (FOLIC ACID)

This water soluble vitamin is helpful for the entire nervous system. It is usually referred to as folic acid. It is thought to work with vitamin B_{12} in the body with amino acid metabolism and with the breaking down of protein into a useable form. And it is known to help stimulate the production of hydrochloric acid which is essential to digestion.

Folic acid is important to the nervous system along with other B-complex vitamins. It is thought to strengthen the nervous system and aid in neurotransmissions.

Folic acid is known to be a component in the production of the genetic cells DNA and RNA. And it aids in healthy tissue growth.

FOLIC ACID AND PREGNANCY

Recent studies have shown that women who take folic acid early in their pregnancies have a greater chance of having babies without certain birth defects. These include neural tube defects such as spina bifida, cleft palate, and anenceplhaly (no brain). Folic acid requirements are much greater during pregnancy. The RDA suggests that a woman during pregnancy consume twice the amount required for normal adults. It seems that folic acid is a crucial element in the development of a healthy fetus. Most experts agree that a well balanced, vitamin supplemented diet is essential for normal growth of the fetus. And certainly a diet rich in folic acid would be wise and beneficial during pregnancy.

Folic acid deficiency is a common vitamin deficiency. When food is overcooked and reheated or improperly stored, most or all of the folic acid can be lost. Many medications such as aspirin can decrease the absorption of folic acid. A supplement is often required.

Folic acid is needed for the absorption of iron and calcium along with vitamin B_{12} and C.

Foods which contain folic acid are green leafy vegetables, beef, lamb, pork, chicken, liver, broccoli, spinach, fresh mushrooms, sprouts, brewer's yeast, eggs, yogurt, whole wheat, vegetables, and carrots.

VITAMIN B_{12} (COBALAMIN)

Vitamin B_{12} is the only vitamin containing a mineral element known as cobalt. It works closely with folic acid to perform functions in the body.

Vitamin B_{12} is important for the metabolism of carbohydrates, fats, and protein. A deficiency can cause many gastrointestinal difficulties.

This vitamin is important to the health of the nervous system. It is thought to be involved with the production of myelin which is a covering of the nerves. And a deficiency may cause emotional problems.

Injections of vitamin B_{12} are sometimes given to individuals suffering from pernicious anemia. But it is important to determine the type of anemia before giving this treatment. A supplement of folic acid when B_{12} is lacking, may cause a more severe deficiency of B_{12}. This type of anemia is seen most often in alcoholics and vegetarians.

Vitamin B_{12} is important for the body's use of amino acids, vitamin D, and in the utilization of iron.

Some studies seem to point to low levels of vitamin B_{12} being a factor in Alzheimer's disease.

Vitamin B_{12} is needed for normal growth, blood cell formation and in healthy skin and mucous membranes.

A deficiency of vitamin B_{12} is rare because relatively little is needed in the body. But those at risk seem to be the elderly, vegetarians, and alcoholics.

Foods which contain vitamin B_{12} include soybeans, wheat germ, liver, kidneys, meat, egg yolk, dairy products, fish, brewer's yeast, pork, almonds, and carrots.

PABA (Para-aminobenzoic Acid)

PABA is essential for the synthesis of folic acid. It is also important for the metabolism of protein in the body. It is an ingredient in many sunscreens and as the ability to prevent sun damage to the skin when applied externally. It is suggested by some to be a preventive to the premature graying of hair.

Sources of PABA are brewer's yeast, liver and wheat germ.

CHOLINE

Choline is thought to be part of the metabolism of fats in the body. It is known to help strengthen the capillaries and lower cholesterol levels in the blood. Choline is essential to nerve function. It aids in the proper distribution of fats in the body and promotes a healthy liver, kidneys, brain and heart. It is needed for the storage of vitamins and minerals especially calcium and vitamin A. It is used to make a neurotransmitter known as acetylcholine which is essential to normal brain function.

Sources of Choline include liver, peas, peanuts, brewer's yeast, fish, wheat germ, egg yolks, sesame seeds, lecithin, and spinach.

INOSITOL

Inositol is thought to help cleanse the blood of excessive fats along with choline. It assists in stimulating the action of the heart and in reducing blood cholesterol levels. It helps to stimulate normal growth patterns and the digestive action.

Inositol is found in liver, soybean, lecithin, oatmeal, molasses, cantaloupe, lima beans, oranges, wheat germ, sesame seeds, whole wheat, and brewer's yeast.

VITAMIN C (ASCORBIC ACID)

This water soluble vitamin is essential to the body. It helps prevent infection by increasing and speeding up activity of white blood cells and aids in destroying viruses and bacteria. It is thought to play a major role in stimulating the immune system and in helping prevent infection and maybe even cancer. Vitamin C in large amounts seems to help produce lymphocytes which are a component of the immune system.Vitamin C is needed by the thymus gland which is involved in the immune system. It is also thought to be able to lessen the length and strength of colds.

GROWTH

Vitamin C is important to the growth of body tissue and in the formation of collagen which is found in connective tissue, bone, and cartilage. It is essential for good teeth, bones and in the growth of children.

Cardiovasular Health

Vitamin C is also thought to be beneficial to the cardiovascular system. It may help prevent high blood pressure and atherosclerosis. And studies seem to show that cholesterol levels are lowered with vitamin C therapy by converting the cholesterol into bile salts. It seems to have the ability to repair arterial walls and prevent cholesterol deposits.

It is essential to the absorption of iron and aids in the storage of folic acid. It is also known to help with the storage of iron in the bone marrow, spleen, and liver. In nature ascorbic acid is found in combination with bioflavonoids. And they are thought to enhance the absorption of vitamin C.

Food sources of vitamin C include broccoli, brussels sprouts, acerola cherry juice, red and green peppers, black currants, collards, turnip greens, parsley, cauliflower, citrus fruits, spinach, papaya, strawberries, and melons.

VITAMIN D (Calciferol)

This important vitamin is responsible for regulating mineral and vitamin metabolism including calcium, phosphorus, and vitamin A. It helps to increase the absorption of calcium and phosphorus. It is produced naturally by the action of sunlight with oils on the skin.

It is important to take vitamin D along with calcium to improve bone strength. The vitamin D aids in the absorption of calcium. This combination is also thought to have some cancer fighting properties.

This vitamin is fat soluble and is stored in the skin, brain, liver, and bones.

Foods rich in vitamin D include dairy products, fish liver oils, egg yolks, spinach, tuna, sardines, and salmon.

VITAMIN E (TOCOPHEROL)

Vitamin E is fat soluble and needed in small amounts. Vitamin A and vitamin E are thought to activate each other. Alpha Tocopherol is the most potent form of vitamin E. Selenium is known to increase the power of vitamin E. And manganese is necessary for vitamin E to be more effective.

It helps control the unsaturated fats in the body and is thought to reduce cholesterol levels in the blood. Vitamin E is also thought to increase the HDL levels in the blood which are a form of cholesterol known to protect against heart disease. It is also used by some to treat circulatory problems.

Vitamin E is used to help in the healing of wounds and in the prevention of scarring. It can be externally applied to surface wounds and scars or taken internally to help prevent internal scar tissue from forming after surgery or injury.

Some studies done link vitamin E to helping reduce fibrocystic breast lumps which are benign cysts on the breast.

Vitamin E is thought to contain properties that protect the body from harmful substances such as toxins and carcinogens. It may help maintain the strength of the cells to combat the development of diseases such as cancer.

Vitamin E is also considered to be a factor in increasing the immune and nervous systems.

Vitamin E is associated with the sex organs. It is though to increase fertility and male potency. It may also help alleviate the symptoms associated with PMS so common with many women.

Vitamin E is found in wheat germ, vegetable oils, peanuts, lettuce, spinach, whole grains, egg yolks, and corn.

VITAMIN F (UNSATURATED FATTY ACIDS)

Vitamin F is fat soluble. It is essential for healthy function of the adrenal and thyroid glands. It is aided in its absorption when taken with vitamin E.

It is found in all unsaturated vegetable oils. It is also found in oats, rye, nuts, avocado, whole raw milk, and cold liver oil.

VITAMIN H (BIOTIN)

Biotin is essential for normal growth of all body tissue and cells. It is helpful in the utilization of B-complex vitamins and is considered to be an essential component of the B-complex. It is not thought of as a true vitamin because it is made in our bodies in the intestines.

It is thought to be helpful in the maintenance of the hair and skin.

Biotin may be helpful in treating nervous system disorders.

Foods which contain this vitamin include brewer's yeast, egg yolks, liver, chicken, pork, lamb, beef, milk, wheat germ, sprouts, molasses, and yogurt.

VITAMIN K

Vitamin K is fat soluble. It is found in some foods that we eat but is also formed in the intestines by bacteria.

It is well known for its blood clotting abilities. It is essential in the formation of prothrombin which is converted into thrombin which is a blood clotting chemical. With vitamin C it is useful to stop bleeding after surgery.

Foods which contain this vitamin are yogurt, spinach, liver, meat, green leafy vegetables, carrots, potatoes, turnips, alfalfa, safflower oil, kelp, whole grains, legumes, and egg yolks.

VITAMIN P (BIOFLAVONOIDS)

Vitamin P increases the effectiveness of vitamin C. The two work together to strengthen connective tissue and capillaries.

It is found in citrus fruits, apricots, blackberries, cherries, grapes, plums, rose hips, buckwheat, and spinach.

VITAMIN T

This vitamin is not very well known. It seems to assist in normalizing blood coagulation and forming of platelets.

It is found in sesame seeds, tahini, and egg yolks.

VITAMIN U

This vitamin was recently discovered. It is high in chlorophyll.

It is found in cabbage juice, sauerkraut, and raw celery juice.

The Importance of Minerals

Many laboratory experiments have been done regarding the importance of minerals in the body and determining what part they play in healthy development. The body certainly needs small amounts of many minerals to function normally. They are sometimes referred to as micronutrients because of the relatively small amounts which are required by the body.These minerals need to be supplied on a daily basis to maintain and regulate necessary body functions. These can either be supplied by a nutritious diet or through supplements. Minerals aid the body in assimilating vitamins. The body needs minerals, vitamins, water, protein, carbohydrates and fats to survive. But minerals can help keep the body young and healthy. They are necessary for the nervous system, normalizing the heartbeat, improving the brain and mental abilities, fighting fatigue and increasing energy, electrolyte balance, and aiding the metabolic process.

Most minerals cannot be used by the body in their free state. They need to be taken in combined form for them to be of benefit to the body. And this combination allows them to be broken down into a more digestible form. This process is called chelation. Minerals may be purchased in chelated form which eliminates the body's need to break them down and makes better use of the minerals.

As the minerals are absorbed into the body, they become a part of the body. They are either used immediately or stored for future use. They help compose the muscles, skin, blood, bone, and cells. But they are mainly stored in the muscle tissue and bone.

Major/trace Minerals

There are two different categories of minerals. These include major minerals or macro minerals and trace minerals or micro minerals. Both are equally important, but the major minerals are those required by the body in large amounts. The trace minerals are only needed in small amounts, and in fact can be toxic if used in large quantities.

Body Fluids

Minerals help regulate the delicate balance of body fluids. They are essential for all mental and physical functions. Minerals aid in the process of osmosis which includes emptying the body of waste and bringing oxygen and nutrients to the cells. They help equalize the fluids in and out of the cells.

It is thought that 28 minerals are found in the human body. 14 of these are considered trace minerals because they are found in such small quantities. Studies are on going as to the part each mineral plays in the body process. The minerals are tested to see what harm a deficit may cause. From the studies done, it appears that iron and iodine are the most important trace minerals. Zinc, copper, manganese, and fluoride are essential to good health. Of lesser importance seem to be molybdenum, selenium, cobalt, nickel, tin, vanadium, and silicon.

Most of the minerals needed by the body can be supplied by the food we eat. Assuming that a proper and nutritious diet is followed. There are some who believe that because of the depletion of nutrients in the soil along with pesticides and food processing, many of the important nutrients are missing from the food we eat. These individuals would promote the use of supplements to achieve the amount of vitamins and minerals needed by the body.

The following are the functions of some of the minerals found in the body.

CALCIUM

Calcium is the most abundant mineral found in the body. And that is a good indicator of just how essential it is. Most of the calcium in the body, approximately 99%, is located in the bones and teeth. The remaining portion is found in the bloodstream and cells.

Calcium is necessary for the transmission of nerve signals. It is important for smooth functioning of the heart muscles and muscular movements of the intestines. And it is best known for its help in maintaining strong and healthy bones. If the body is lacking in calcium, it will fill the deficit by reaching into supplies found in the bones. When this condition continues over a period of time, loss of bone mass can occur and cause brittle bones as well as osteoporosis.

Studies have been done confirming the importance of adequate amounts of calcium in the body. Calcium supplements seem to help reduce the incidence of high blood pressure. And studies have confirmed the importance of calcium in helping to prevent colon cancer.

To function efficiently calcium must be in combination with magnesium, phosphorus, vitamins A, C, and D as well as zinc. These nutrients help the body to absorb and make proper use of calcium.

Foods rich in calcium include dairy products, collard greens, barley, kale, nuts, cereals, sesame seeds, most green vegetables and whole grains.

PHOSPHORUS

This mineral has many important functions in the body. It is the second most abundant mineral found in the body. Phosphorus is found mainly in the bones and teeth. The rest is located throughout the body in the fluids, blood, and cells.

Phosphorus and Calcium work together. It helps with the formation of strong bones and teeth, aids the pH balance of the blood, helps metabolize fats, aids in activating the oxidation of carbohydrates, and is required for the production of body energy. Phosphorus combines with fats in the blood and is then known as phospholipids. The phospholipids have an important role. They become part of the cell structure which regulates the movement of material in and out of the cells.

For phosphorus to be absorbed and utilized by the body, calcium and vitamin D are required. Phosphorus and calcium levels are closely linked. They both work together in many important functions.

Foods rich in phosphorus include dairy products, nuts, beans, whole grains, fish, poultry, meat, eggs, pumpkin seeds, dark green leafy vegetables, barley, and rice bran.

POTASSIUM

Potassium works with sodium to regulate fluids and the flow of nutrients in and out of the cells. The cells actually contain more potassium than any other mineral found in the body.

It is involved in the maintenance of regular heart rhythm. It helps stimulate the kidneys and helps with normal function of the adrenals. It is important in stimulating the nerve impulses which cause muscle contraction.

Potassium is responsible for helping convert glucose into glycogen to be stored in the body. Deficiencies in potassium can cause muscle weakness, muscle spasms, heart problems, nausea, and vomiting.

Potassium is found in some dairy products, fish, meat, poultry, legumes, whole grains, bananas and most fruits, vegetables including bitter greens, and almonds.

SODIUM

Most of the sodium in the body is found in the fluid surrounding the cells. Sodium works with chlorine to regulate the pH of the fluids in the body. Potassium and sodium work together to regulate the flow of nutrients in and out of the cells.

Excess sodium can cause serious health problems including hypertension and edema. It is a valuable mineral but can usually be supplied in the foods we eat without a supplement.

Foods which contain sodium include shellfish, carrots, beets, artichokes, dried beef, watercress, and almost all food.

CHLORINE

Chlorine is essential for the production of vital gastric juices aiding in digestion. It must be present for the body to manufacture hydrochloric acid which is part of the digestion process and necessary for the liver to help eliminate waste. It is needed to help regulate the pH balance of the blood in very small trace amounts.

Chlorine easily combines with other minerals and chemicals. Because of this, it may be harmful to some substances. It is thought to destroy vitamin E which has many important functions.

It is rarely lacking in the diet because of the chlorination of drinking water.

Sources of chlorine include drinking water, sea greens, olives, salt, fish, rye flour, and sardines.

IRON

Iron is a mineral that most people are familiar with. Yet many people suffer from a deficit of iron in their diets. Iron is found in all the cells of the body. Most is located in the red blood cells and is essential to the process of carrying oxygen to all parts of the body. Iron is a major component of hemoglobin. And hemoglobin is what makes red blood cells and carries the oxygen. Iron is also found in myogloben which is a red pigment found in the muscles and is needed for electron transport.

Iron is not easily absorbed by the body. For proper assimilation, an adequate amount of hydrochloric acid must be present in the stomach and vitamins C and E, calcium and copper. These will enhance the function of iron.

Iron is known as the anti-anemia mineral because of its aid in the oxygenating of cells and combining with protein to form hemoglobin. Anemia occurs when the hemoglobin levels are low and the tissues in the body become oxygen deficient. Iron deficiency symptoms include, fatigue, pale coloring, and heart palpitations.

Iron is thought to play a part in aiding the immune system in fighting disease. Low levels of iron can make the body more susceptible to disease and infection.

Iron is the most difficult mineral to provide for the body. And iron deficiency is the most common deficiency problem throughout the world. Therefore, a supplement is usually needed.

Foods rich in iron include liver, greens, spinach, blackberries, cherries, dried fruits, raw egg yolks, meat, fish, whole grain bread, potatoes, and leafy vegetables.

MANGANESE

This is a trace mineral essential for proper function of the pituitary gland as well as the healthy function of all the body's glands. It is found in many enzymes in the body and is important in helping metabolize fats, protein and energy. It aids in the utilization of glucose. It also helps in reproduction and in normal functioning of the central nervous system.

There have been studies done which indicate that a diet deficient in manganese may play a role in some birth defects. And manganese is thought to be helpful in improving the immune system.

Manganese is lacking in most refined foods and a supplement is usually recommended.

Food sources of manganese include nuts, seeds, avocado, whole grains, barley, kidney beans, eggs, leaf lettuce, grapefruit, and apricots.

MAGNESIUM

Magnesium is essential to the body. About half of the magnesium is located in the bones. It is required for proper growth and health of the bones and teeth along with phosphorus and calcium.

Magnesium is an essential part of the enzyme system which carries elements through the cell membranes. It is a major regulator of cellular activity including the maintenance of DNA and RNA. It is considered an anti-stress mineral. And studies have found that low magnesium levels may be associated with depression, delirium, and other mental disturbances.

Magnesium works to improve the muscular tone of the blood vessels along with sodium, potassium, and calcium. This is why magnesium may be an important contributor to preventing diseases associated with the blood vessels.

It assists in the absorption of calcium, phosphorous, sodium, potassium, and vitamin B-complex, C and E.

Foods rich in magnesium include dairy products, brown rice, wheat germ, corn meal, almonds, avocados, whole grains, greens, berries, barley, meat, fish, nuts, blackstrap molasses, and seeds.

IODINE

Iodine is a trace mineral needed only in very small amounts. It is part of the thyroid hormones thyroxine and triodothyronine. The majority is located in the thyroid gland and the rest is found throughout the body mainly in the fluid surrounding the cells.

Iodine is a part of the proper functioning of the thyroid. It helps to regulate metabolism, influence growth, regulation of the nervous and muscular systems, and in helping the body assimilate nutrients.

Goiter is a condition in which the thyroid gland becomes enlarged. It is a symptom of iodine deficiency.

Food sources of iodine include, table salt, seafood, seaweed, garlic, onions, and eggplant.

FLUORINE

This is considered an essential trace mineral, but it has been the subject of much controversy because of its presence as an additive to drinking water in many states. The fluorine added to drinking water is usually in the form of sodium fluoride, sodium silicon fluoride, or hydro fluorosilic acid which are not natural sources and have caused some contention.

Fluorine is known to increase the absorption of calcium to create stronger bones and teeth.

Food sources of fluorine include seafood, milk, egg yolks and some water.

COPPER

Copper is an important trace mineral. It is stored in the liver, brain, heart and kidneys.

It aids in the absorption of calcium, the assimilation of iron and the formation of red blood cells. Copper aids in taste sensitivity. It is part of every body tissue. It helps the body oxidize vitamin C. Though needed in only small amounts, copper is thought to help the immune system.

Deficiencies of copper are rare. But individuals who are lacking in other nutrients, may also lack copper.

Food sources of copper include liver, whole grains, almonds, legumes, nuts, shellfish, meats, raisins, beans, and blackstrap molasses.

COBALT

This trace mineral is essential for human nutrition. It aids in the assimilation and synthesis of vitamin B_{12} and stimulates many enzymes in the body. It is actually a component of vitamin B_{12}. It aids in the building of red blood cells.

The amount of cobalt needed by the body is small. And a lack or excess are both detrimental. A lack can lead to pernicious anemia and an excess is thought to cause an enlarged thyroid.

Cobalt is present in all animal and most dairy products. It is also found in sea foods, apricots, oysters, clams, and sea vegetation.

CHROMIUM

Chromium is a less known trace mineral but equally important. It is essential for the synthesis of fatty acids and the metabolism of glucose for energy. It is also known to increase the efficiency of insulin by aiding in the supply of glucose to every cell. It helps regulate blood sugar levels.

Food containing chromium include brewer's yeast, sugar beets, whole grains, corn oil and clams.

ZINC

This trace mineral performs many vital body functions. It helps with the absorption of vitamins in the body. The body does not keep a supply of zinc. Some is stored in the bones but it is not thought to be available for use by other areas of the body. It is needed by the body on a daily basis and needs to be supplied.

Zinc aids in the synthesis of RNA and DNA which are important for cell division and growth. It helps with reproductive function.

It helps form skin, hair and nails. And it is thought to help in the healing process of wounds and burns. Zinc is thought to be a component of over 20 enzymes found in the body. It is an essential part of many enzymes involved in digestion and metabolism. Zinc is essential to the growth process.

The highest concentrations of zinc are found in the eye. Zinc seems to be involved with vitamin A in aiding with night vision.

Vitamin A must be present for zinc to be properly absorbed by the body.

Food sources of zinc include meats, poultry, fish, seafood, liver, eggs, legumes, whole grains, wheat germ, pumpkin seeds, avocado, and asparagus.

SELENIUM

This is considered a relatively new trace mineral but is accepted as essential. Selenium is present in all body tissues but is found mainly in the kidneys, liver, spleen, pancreas, and testes.

It is a helper to other nutrients especially vitamin E. It helps the body utilize oxygen and assists in the normal growth function. It may help prevent chromosome breakage which causes birth defects.

Low selenium levels have been associated with mental deficiencies, rheumatoid arthritis, and even cancer. It seems to play a role as an antioxidant and anticancer mineral. Free radicals cause damage to the cells and may lead to cancer. Selenium is a part of the enzyme glutathione peroxidase which has the ability to protect the cells from damage. Studies have been conducted which seem to point to the ability of selenium to prevent cancer in animals.

Food sources of selenium include meat, seafood, bran, whole grains, tuna fish, broccoli, onions, asparagus, mushrooms, and tomatoes.

SULPHUR

Sulphur is known to purify and tone the body. It is not considered deficient in the diet because of its concentration in protein. It is involved in collagen formation which helps maintain healthy hair, fingernails and skin. It is an essential component of some amino acids. It is found inside of all the cells in the body. Sulphur is thought to work with the B-complex vitamins.

Garlic and onions have sulphur compounds. This is thought to be part of the reason for their odor.

Foods which contain sulphur include kale, cabbage, cauliflower, brussels sprouts, watercress, parsley, celery, fish, eggs, and nuts.

VANADIUM

Vanadium is not known to be essential to existence. But it is contained in the body tissue and is excreted in the urine. So it is thought to play a role in the life process.

Some believe that this trace mineral may aid in preventing cardiovascular disease. And it is known to lower serum cholesterol levels. There is not much information available but it is thought to be a factor in normal growth. It is associated with iron metabolism. And it is thought to help in the growth and health of bone, cartilage and teeth.

Foods which contain vanadium include black pepper, fish, seafood, liver, soybeans, corn, olive oil, and meat.

MOLYBDENUM

Molybdenum is a part of some enzymes. It is found in all tissues, skin, liver and kidneys. It helps with the mobilization of iron. It is thought to inhibit dental carries. Some feel that molybdenum may help in reducing esophageal cancer.

Good food sources of molybdenum include buckwheat, lima beans, barley, wheat germ, meat, legumes, liver, and green leafy vegetables.

NICKEL

Nickel is a trace mineral but there is quite a bit present in the body. There is relatively little known about this mineral. But it is believed to aid in membrane metabolism and nucleic acid stabilization. Nickel helps activate some enzymes. It can be extremely toxic. And it is present in cigarette smoke. A nutritionally sound diet is rarely deficient in nickel.

Sources of nickel include tea, cocoa, gelatin, and kidney beans.

TIN

It is thought to be necessary but it is not agreed upon as to how it actually works. It is used in some medicines. Tin is thought to function with iron and copper. Toothpastes containing stannous fluoride contain tin.

SILICON

Silicon is important to normal growth and bone development. It is found abundantly in the soil. Silicon combined with oxygen forms rocks. It is found in small amounts in the bones and teeth. It aids in forming cartilage.

ALUMINUM

This trace mineral is found in the body but can be extremely toxic. It seems to help with the activity of some enzymes but is only needed in trace amounts. It may play a role in protein synthesis. When aluminum utensils are used in cooking, aluminum may be absorbed in the body. It is thought by some to be a factor in Alzheimer's disease.

CADMIUM

Cadmium is also a toxic trace mineral. It is thought that it will take the place of zinc in the body if zinc is lacking in the diet. Cigarette smoke contains cadmium and is known to cause emphysema. It is thought to contribute to high blood pressure and cardiovascular disease. Cadmium is found in coffee, tea, refined foods, and some water supplies.

LEAD

Lead can be very toxic. It causes many different problems known as lead poisoning. Smoking and smog are sources of lead and can lead to problems. Excess lead accumulation can be from leaded gasoline, exhaust, leaded paint, and some cosmetics.

MERCURY

Another toxic trace mineral is mercury. It is found in lakes and streams due to waste dumping from manufacturing companies. Fish are often sources of mercury poisoning as their natural habitat is polluted. Mercury poisoning can cause birth and genetic defects.

Food Combining

There are many health advocates who follow strict methods of food combinations in their diets. Some experts believe in the theory and others don't. The basic theory is that too many different foods eaten at on time may cause heartburn, poor absorption, improper digestion, fermentation, gas, and the formation of toxins. They believe that simple preparation of food will help digestion, assimilation, and elimination.

A glass of water with half a lemon squeezed is recommended first thing in the morning. This is used to clean the stomach and help the liver to begin functioning. Fresh fruit, cereal, seeds, or nuts are suggested as breakfast foods. Fresh vegetable salad, nuts, vegetables, and rice are encouraged for lunch. And for dinner a salad, steamed vegetable and baked potato are thought to be the right combination.

Individuals who use food combining suggest eating no protein after two o'clock P.M. It is harder for the body to digest protein in the evening and may cause fermentation.

Guidelines for Food Combining

Louise Tenney, in her book NUTRITIONAL GUIDE WITH FOOD COMBINING published by Woodland Books, 1991 on page 41, lists the following guidelines for healthy eating and proper food combining.

"1. Eat acids and starches at separate meals
2. Eat protein foods and carbohydrate foods at separate meals.
3. Eat but one concentrated protein food at a meal.
4. Eat proteins and acids at separate meals.
5. Eat fats and proteins at separate meals.
6. Eat sugars and proteins at separate meals.
7. Eat starches and sugars at separate meals."

Protein and starch foods are not recommended to be eaten together. But in nature these two are combined in grains, seeds, and vegetables in a way that they are digestible. When proteins and starches are eaten together, they do not seem to be assimilated well. Proteins require an acid medium for digestion.

Carbohydrates need an alkaline medium for digestion. Food combiners feel that an improper food combination will upset the digestive system and cause gas, bloating and lethargy.

Foods high in protein and grains are thought to be acid forming foods. It is usually recommend that alkaline to acid foods should be eaten in a four to one ratio. Alkaline foods include vegetables, most fruits, and almonds. Foods which are acid forming are animal proteins (meat, shellfish, fish, eggs, cheese, poultry, nuts (except almonds), and foods made from cereal starches and sugar.

Most individuals in the nutritional field suggest that milk products should be eaten alone.

DIGESTION TIME

The digestion time of different foods depends on how easily they are to assimilate in the body.

Green Vegetables	5 hours
Raw Juices	15 minutes
Fat	12 hours
Protein (meat)	12 hours
Protein (fat)	12 hours
Starch	5 hours
Fruit, sweet, dried	3 hours
Fruit (acid)	2 hours
Fruit, fresh, sweet	3 hours
Melon	2 hours
Sugar	2 hours
Milk	12 hours

Juicing

Juicing has become very popular in the past few years. Books are being written and even television shows have been devoted solely to promoting different methods of juicing. What has brought all this excitement about juices into the public eye? And are there really benefits?

BENEFITS OF JUICING

Advocates of juicing swear by the possibilities and benefits. Stephen Blauer, in his book entitled THE JUICING BOOK published by Avery Pub. Group Inc. on page ix, states, "Fresh juice is more than an excellent source of vitamins, minerals, enzymes, purified water, proteins, carbohydrates, and chlorophyll. Because it is in liquid form, fresh juice supplies nutrition that is not wasted to fuel its own digestion as it is with whole fruits, vegetables, and grasses. As a result, the body can quickly and easily make maximum use of all the nutrition that fresh juice offers."

ADVANTAGES OF FRESH JUICES

The key is that most juices bought in the grocery store are not fresh. They may be made from concentrates and not the whole fruit. These are not as nutritionally beneficial as fresh juice. Some of the vitamins and minerals are lost in the processing. And then there is the problem with additives. Many do not have additives, but some contain preservatives, added sugar, and food coloring. Pesticides used on produce is also a consideration. Some pesticides banned from the United States are used by foreign countries. And they sometimes find their way back into our food.

DISADVANTAGES OF PREPACKAGED JUICES

Cerie Calbom and Maureen Keane in their book JUICING FOR LIFE published by Avery Pub. Group Inc. on page 22 state, "Fruits and vegetables take a lot of abuse before they enter a bottle or can. Often, chemicals are poured on them for a variety of reasons. Chemicals can destroy nutrients, and when chemicals are washed off with lots of water, minerals are leached out. Some chemical residues will be left behind for your body to process. Moreover, many juices are heated to high temperatures as a part of pasteurization, which prolongs shelf life. This process kills enzymes, the spark plugs of life. Often, additives like sodium benzoate, benzoic acid, sodium nitrate, BHA, and BHT are added. Then the juices go to warehouses, where they may sit for weeks or months before reaching your store. By the time processed juices get to you, most of the nutrients have been lost. But when you make fresh juice, you're assured of getting a large proportion of nutrients present in the raw fruits and vegetables."

Vitamin and mineral supplements can be effective. But many are synthetically produced and hard for the body to assimilate. Using natural juices, the vitamins and minerals can be taken in their original form. They are natural and easy for the body to assimilate.

Fresh juices are easy to prepare. And they can be much more tasty and nutritious then the fruit or vegetable alone. Many people who juice, feel that they have improved their overall health.

Many individuals who juice regularly feel that juicing can supply the body with the nutrients it needs. Juicing the fruits and vegetables makes the body's job easier. The digestion process naturally juices the food we eat. And many believe that large amounts of fruits and vegetables are needed to fill the body's nutritional needs. But the body cannot handle too much bulk and fiber. So juicing can supply nutrients without extreme amounts of bulk.

FIBER

Fiber is very important. And juicing advocates advise eating fruits, vegetables, and whole grains along with the juice diet.

Some feel that because of modern farming techniques now practiced, many of the nutrients are lost in the process. These nutrient depleting procedures include chemical fertilizers, pesticides and the actual food processing. Because of the nutrients lost, many feel that more food is needed to actually meet the needs of the body.

GUIDELINES

GENERAL GUIDELINES FOR JUICING:

1. Try and use organically grown produce whenever possible. Remember to peel or scrub fruit before using.
2. Wash all produce thoroughly before using. They can be scrubbed with a vegetable brush. Cut off bruises or moldy sections which may contain toxins or undesirable tastes.
3. The pits found in fruits such as peaches, plums and avocados should be removed. Seeds in oranges, limes, lemons, grapes, etc. can be juiced. Apple seeds should be removed because of the small amounts of cyanide they contain. but some use the apple seeds without any problems.
4. Oranges, grapefruits and bananas along with waxed fruits should be peeled.
5. Fruits and vegetables should generally be sliced before being put in the juicer. Check with the instructions that accompany your particular juicer.

6. Bananas and avocados should not be put in the juicer alone. They do not contain enough natural juice. Add them to other juices slowly.
7. Use ripe fruit and vegetables. They are the most beneficial to the body because they contain the most nutrients.
8. Most fruits and vegetables should be juiced raw. Some hard vegetables should be lightly steamed and cooled first including broccoli, cauliflower, potatoes, etc.
9. Do not mix fruits and vegetables. The acids in fruit are thought to turn the vegetable oils rancid. Apples are the exception.

Juices as Medicine

Generally, juices are not considered medicine. But because of the high concentration of vitamins and minerals, many use them to help in building the immune system and in helping the body to heal itself when faced with an illness.

Fresh juices are full of pure nutrition. They contain many different nutrients including beta carotene, vitamin C, vitamin E. minerals, and enzymes. Many studies done have pointed to the use of vitamins and minerals in prevention and healing. Beta carotene has been been acclaimed as aiding in the treatment of some forms of cancer. Vitamins C and E, are thought to help in the prevention of cancer and in building the immune system. And the B-complex vitamins are known to build the nervous system and help aid in stress and in the prevention of stress related illnesses.

Recommended Juice Remedies

Juicing advocates emphasize the juices most important for the body. These include carrot, celery, dark green leafy vegetables, melons, apples, and citrus fruits. The following are some specific juices recommended for some illnesses.

1. Common Cold:
   Carrot, Parsley, Spinach
   Grapefruit, Lemon, Pineapple

2. Acne:
   Papaya
   Carrot, Green Pepper, Parsley

3. Heart Disease:
   Vegetable Greens
   Garlic, Onion

4. Indigestion:
   Papaya, Lemon, Ginger
   Cabbage, Celery

5. Stress:
   Broccoli, Red Pepper, Parsley, Carrot
   Cantaloupe, Ginger

There are many books on the market which contain excellent recipes for juicing. The variety is unlimited. And many recipes are fun and easy to make and excellent for all members of the family.

Exercise

INTRODUCTION

It is common knowledge that exercise is extremely important. It is an essential part of total body health. But studies continue to show that the majority of Americans live sedentary lives. They do not participate in regular exercise. Children today are less fit and weigh more than they did 30 years ago. They spend much of their free time in front of the television. But these statistics need to change and adults as well as children need to become more active.

LESS ACTIVE LIFESTYLES TODAY

Physical demands on man have changed. We have many energy saving devises that make life easier. But with these great inventions, our health has suffered. Automobiles take us where we want to go. The dish washer and washing machines help us save time and use less physical energy. We aren't required to work the land in order to eat. We can drive to the super market and pick out fresh produce all year. And with less physical demands on our bodies, we are less fit. And regular exercise is needed in order to keep the body in shape.

EXERCISE BENEFITS

The benefits from exercise are many. A fit body is more efficient. Studies show that physical inactivity can lead to serious health problems. And some believe that a lack of exercise is responsible for many of today's health problems. Coronary heart disease, high blood pressure, high blood cholesterol levels, hypertension, strokes, and even cancer are associated in part to a lack of exercise.

Colon Cancer Rates

In the March 1992 issue of AMERICAN HEALTH magazine an article written by Paul McCarthy was published stating that regular exercise can help prevent colon cancer."Most recently, a team of researchers headed by I-Min Lee, a research associate in epidemiology at Harvard University's School of Public Health, reviewed the exercise habits of 17,000 male Harvard alumni who are part of a survey begun in 1962. They found those who burned 1,000 calories or more per week through exercise were half as likely to contract colon cancer as those who didn't.

Other studies have produced similar results. A survey of nearly 3,000 men of scientists at the University of Southern California School of Medicine found those who did sedentary work had a 60% higher colon cancer rate than men who had physically active jobs. And in a 19-year study of more than one million Swedish men, published in 1986, those who sat for more than half their working hours were found to be 30% likelier to get colon cancer than the men who spent less than 20 % of their time seated.

Why does physical activity reduce colon cancer risk? The most popular theory, says Lee, "is that when people exercise, food passes through the gut faster, minimizing the colon's exposure to any carcinogens."

Immune System

Scientists also speculate that exercise may enhance the immune system. If so, exercise might prevent other cancers too. In one of the few studies done in this area, Rose Frisch, an associate professor of population sciences at the Harvard School of Public Health, compared female former college athletes with their classmates—5,400 subjects in all. Frisch and her colleagues found the non-athletes had 2 1/2 times as many reproductive-system cancers and twice as many breast cancers as their more active classmates. "This was moderate exercise," says Frisch, "not Olympic-level training."

Physical Examination Before Starting

Before beginning an exercise program, it is important to have a thorough medical examination if there is any doubt as to your health. Some may require in depth heart testing to determine problems that may exist. Exercise is important to health and most people can participate in a moderate exercise program without any problems.

Regular, Moderate Exercise

Regular, moderate exercise is important to good health. Experts agree that exercise can increase circulation, increase the digestive process, strengthen the heart, reduce blood pressure, increase lung capacity and oxygen utilization, lower blood cholesterol levels, and promote an overall sense of well-being due in part to the release of endorphins. It also helps cleanse the body through perspiration, tone the nervous system, and strengthen the immune system to prevent disease.

More Activity in Our Lifestyles

Becoming more active is an important part of health. One important step is to use our bodies more. Take the stairs whenever possible instead of the elevator or escalator, park a few blocks away from an appointment and walk, put more energy into housework, walk or ride a bike to activities, and spend time working in the yard are a few suggestions.

A regular exercise program is needed to keep the body in optimum condition. Experts usually suggest a minimum of 20 to 30 minutes three to five times per week. But it is a good idea to try and do some type of activity to increase the heart rate each day. It is important to start out slow and gradually increase activity. Doing too much in the beginning can cause pain and injury which may discourage and end exercise routines.

Aerobic Exercise

Aerobic exercise is important to fitness. These are the activities that create a training effect. Aerobic means with oxygen and activities which increase the breathing and heart rate for an extended period of time. They improve the ability of the heart and lungs through regular exercise.There are many different activities which are considered aerobic. Anaerobic means without oxygen. These activities are those that require quick action and bursts of energy and oxygen such as sprinting and are not continuous over a period of time.

Heart Rate

It is important to monitor the heart rate when beginning an exercise program. There are different formulas to calculate maximum heart rate levels. This simple formula is recommended by the Institute of Aerobic Research. It is 220 minus your age to predict maximum heart rate. For men in great condition it is 205 minus half your age. Aerobic exercise should work at 75 to 80 % of the maximum heart rate. The heart rate can be checked by placing the fingers on the artery of the neck.

I usually don't worry about my heart rate while I am exercising. I can tell how hard I am working by how I feel. I perspire and breath hard but am able to carry on a conversation. If I am hurting, I slow down. If I am out of breath,

I slow down. Learn to listen to your body and don't push too hard.

Warm up Cool down

A warm up period is important to prepare the body for a work out. This should include a slow version of whatever activity you are doing. For instance, if you are running, start out slow for the first three minutes and gradually work into a faster pace. In addition, a cool down is also important. Don't stop exercising abruptly. Take some time to gradually slow down. The body needs time to adjust and the blood pressure should come down gradually as to do the most good. Slow down for approximately five minutes before ending an exercise period.

Exercise should be enjoyable. Pick activities that are fun for you. Music can also help relax and make exercise enjoyable. Turn on the music when exercising at home, or wear headphones outside to run or walk.

There are many different activities to choose from that will increase endurance and promote body fitness. The following are a few suggestions.

WALKING

Walking is probably the easiest activity you can do. All that is required is a good pair of walking shoes and yourself. And it is an exercise that can be done by almost everyone. It can be done in just about any location and at anytime. Walking is considered to be safe, convenient, and very beneficial. Experts suggest working up to walking three miles in approximately 45 minutes four to five days a week. But for individuals who are out of shape, beginning with a brisk walk for 15 minutes is recommended and gradually adding time.

A brisk pace is needed for aerobic benefits, but even a casual stroll can be beneficial. It is important to concentrate on good posture while walking. Relax the neck and shoulders but keep the head high. The heel should touch the ground first with the weight coming gradually across the foot.

To make walking more challenging, pick up the pace, add hand weights, or do some hill walking. And to cure boredom, wear some headphones and listen to music or change the normal path you follow. Walk in different directions and explore new areas.

Just being in the out of doors is a reward in itself. Enjoy the changing of the seasons. Breath the fresh air. Explore new territory. There is a feeling of resurgence from spending time with nature and learning to value the beauty of the world in which we live.

RUNNING/ JOGGING

Running became popular with the exercise craze of the eighties. But many have suffered stress injuries related to the impact on the joints and muscles. Consequently, many of the runners of the eighties, including myself, have chosen walking instead.

Running does have its benefits. It can be very intense and promote fitness quickly. Running and jogging are known to help condition individuals and also to help burn fat and calories at a quicker pace. Running also releases endorphins which create a feeling of well-being. This is sometimes referred to as a runner's high.

To help prevent injuries, it helps to run on a flat surface. Most people run on the roads and sidewalks which are made of concrete and can be very stressful on the joints. Asphalt is also stressful, but not as bad as concrete. If possible, run on the grass or any soft surface to avoid injury. Indoor tracks offer a nice, soft, and flexible surface for jogging or running. They are built with a cushioning affect which helps soften the stress.

Correct running shoes are very important. Choose a shoe that fits well and has some cushioning. These can help control and minimize injuries by absorbing some of the shock sustained by running.

Be sure to pay attention to your body. It is important to be aware of problems that may develop. Stress on the knee joints, back, hips and ankles can cause injury. If you feel pain or discomfort, lay off for a few days and start back gradually. If problems continue, another type of aerobic exercise may be more appropriate and just as beneficial.

CYCLING

Bicycling is ever increasing in popularity. People are using their bikes as a form of transportation rather than just a recreational tool. And it is an excellent source of aerobic exercise. It is much less stressful on the joints. And people with knee injuries often prefer this type of exercise.

It is important to choose a bike that is the right size and type. There are a wide range available with many different purposes. And they range a great deal in price and quality. A well recommended bike shop has trained sales people that can aid you when making a choice on the correct bike to purchase.

I prefer the mountain bike type which allows you to ride off the road, is sturdy, and sits upright with less strain on the back. A good comfortable seat makes riding more enjoyable.

When cycling, it is important to be careful about where you ride. There is a certain danger associated with motor vehicles when riding on congested roads. Cycling can be most enjoyed on paths or quiet roads. The natural beauty may be observed without the distractions and fumes when automobiles are around.

Stationary bikes can also be used. Especially when the weather is bad. Many recreation centers and health clubs have stationary bikes.

AEROBIC DANCING

Aerobic dance has become one of the country's most popular forms of exercise. Music and friends help make this an attractive option. And this form of exercise can be very beneficial as well as a lot of fun.

This type of dance class usually consists of a warm-up, exercise, dance routines, and cool-down. The routines usually follow simple dance movements and are lead by an instructor.

Aerobic dance classes are usually available at local recreation centers as well as health clubs. Classes are generally available at different levels of ability and it is in your best interest to choose one that specifically matches your level of fitness. There are usually classes offered involving low-impact aerobics which minimize the stress on the joints and are less susceptible to injury. These offer softer routines without a lot of the jarring and jumping movements. The arms are used more during the low-impact to insure that the heart be up at the target rate selected for each individual.

Good aerobics shoes are necessary to help lessen the chance of serious injury. And the dancing surface should be a hardwood floor preferably with spring suspension under. Concrete and thick carpet can be dangerous and are highly discouraged.

SWIMMING

Swimming is enjoyed by many. And those who swim, are usually very enthusiastic about the benefits. It is not as convenient as many aerobic activities, but it fills the needs of many individuals.

In the water, there is a freedom of movement. For people suffering from injuries, this can allow them to exercise without furthering the damage while aiding in the healing. It can be very invigorating without putting stress on the joints.

Swimming is a sport that exercises the entire body. The arms, chest, hips, and legs are all used. The swimming motion also helps stretch the muscles while exercising them. Swimming does not produce the same aerobic conditioning as seen in running and walking. But it also does not put the same amount of stress on the body which is important for some individuals. The freestyle or crawl stroke is thought to be the most effective for fitness.

Studies have shown that swimming does not produce the same degree of fat burning capabilities as other aerobic activities. But it is still a beneficial form of exercise. And some choose to combine swimming with other forms of aerobic exercise alternating swimming and jogging, for instance.

OTHER WATER EXERCISE

Water exercise and aerobics classes are available at some health clubs and recreation centers. These usually are a combination of dance, strokes, and exercise. They can be a lot of fun and more interesting than lap swimming.

Some people have problems with the chlorine in pools. Often the chlorine is not distributed evenly or too much is added. Most of the problems occur soon after the chlorine is added. Knowing what times this occurs can relieve some of the problems. A good pair of goggles are essential to protect the eyes from irritation.

CROSS-COUNTRY SKIING

This activity is considered to be the very best for aerobic exercise. It is very intense and works a wide range of muscle groups. Injury is minimal and it is an excellent aerobic conditioner. Every part of the body can get a work out. The body does not receive jarring movements but the movements are smooth and rhythmic.

But, unfortunately this sport is seasonal and only available in certain locations. Equipment must be maintained and some skill is necessary. There are indoor machines available that are similar to cross country skiing and basically use the same muscles and produce a good cardiovascular conditioning.

JUMPING ROPE

Jumping rope is easy and can be done just about anywhere. It is inexpensive and can be done in all types of weather. Athletes often use the jump rope in their training to improve coordination and cardiovascular fitness. Once a routine and rhythm are sustained, it can be enjoyable, soothing, and very beneficial on the body.

Good athletic shoes are important to absorb some of the shock on the joints. Correct posture is important. Keep the head up and relaxed. The back should be straight and knees bent. The wrists should control the motion of the rope. A dance motion can be used alternating feet instead of jumping with both feet together.

STAIR CLIMBING

Walking up stairs can help with the body fitness. And many stair stepping machines are available. Stepping at a slow pace can still produce a training effect. The requirement is a steady motion continuous for at least fifteen to thirty minutes.

MINI-TRAMPOLINE

This is a favorite of many health conscious people. It is also known as rebounding. It is known to create a cardiovascular fitness as well as coordination. It can be done just about anywhere and the mini-tramps are easily transported. You can jog, jump, or do dance movements. Be careful when first starting out. It is advisable to hang on to a railing or chair while bouncing when beginning.

OTHER SPORTS

Activities such as soccer, basketball, football, baseball, and tennis are a lot of fun. But they all involve amounts of starting and stopping. They can produce some beneficial effects, but to insure fitness training activities that require a constant steady movement are important.

GENERAL RECOMMENDATIONS

GENERAL RECOMMENDATIONS FOR AEROBIC EXERCISE:

1. Become more active. Take the stairs, walk, park farther away from appointments, and put more energy into all activities.
2. Start out gradual. Don't try and do to much too quickly.
3. Warm-up by doing a slow version of activity chosen.
4. Cool-down at the end of an activity.
5. Check with a medical professional before beginning.
6. Listen to your body. If you hurt, stop.

7. Don't exercise while you are sick.
8. Make exercising a habit!
9. Learn to enjoy exercise.

Two Examples of Alternative Health Techniques

The following are two common problems facing most of us today, stress and weight control, and natural approachs to solving them.

Stress Relief

Life is stressful. In fact, every individual whether they choose to interact with others or live a solitary life, must deal with stress on a regular basis. But stress is not always bad. It can motivate and challenge us to perform seemingly impossible tasks. Since there is no way to avoid confronting difficult situations, it is important to learn to deal with them in a positive way.

Stressful situations can build up over the years and take a toll on physical as well as emotional health. Stress can be controlled by improving our ability to cope with situations that cause tension.

INTERNAL AND EXTERNAL

Stress includes both internal and external pressure. Usually an external stress causes us to internalize the problem agitating our minds and bodies by affecting the nervous system and creating stress related illnesses. External stress is present continually. This may include other people, traffic, bills, noise, etc. But how we react to these stresses, affects our internal emotions. And these emotions can actually lead to serious physical illness.

Some external detrimental situations can be changed. But more often than not, external stresses need to be confronted. Situations that include abuse and destructive relationships must be changed.

There have been many studies done that establish a correlation between emotional and physical ailments. The nervous system and the immune system are connected. One study conducted by a group of researchers in Wisconsin reveals this information. ("Specific Attitudes in Initial Interviews with Patients Having Different Psychosomatic Diseases", by Dr. David T. Graham, M.D., Psychosomatic Medicine, Vol. XXIV, No. 3.) Their results indicate the following correlations:

DISEASE: STRESSFUL CONDITION REPORT

ACNE: A feeling of being nagged or picked on, accompanied by a desire to be left alone.

BRONCHIAL ASTHMA: Feeling rejected and unloved; wanting to shut out the rejecting person or situation.

CONSTIPATION: A feeling of being trapped in a negative situation, when there is no way to change.

DUODENAL ULCERS: Feeling unjustly treated, and wanting to take revenge.

ECZEMA: Feeling thwarted and misunderstood, with no alternative but to take out such frustrations on oneself.

HIVES: Having a sense of taking an unfair beating, and being unable to do anything about it.

HYPERTENSION: Feeling constantly endangered.

HYPERTHYROIDISM: (overactive thyroid gland), fear of losing a loved one, or loved object.

LOW BACKACHE: Wanting to run away, to escape from an unpleasant situation.

METABOLIC EDEMA: (Fluid retention by the body's tissues), a sense of being unduly burdened, and of wanting others to carry their share of the load.

MIGRAINES: Feeling driven toward the achievement of some goal or goals; can relax only after the completion of such goals.

PSORIASIS: A constant sensation of gnawing irritation that has to be put up with.

RAYNAUD'S DISEASE: (Chronic constriction and spasms of blood vessels of the toes, fingers, tip of nose, etc.) a feeling of hostility.

RHEUMATOID ARTHRITIS: (A specific type of arthritis involving inflammation of the joints resembling symptoms of rheumatism), feeling constrained and restricted.

VOMITING: Guilt for some wrong doing on the patient's past.

The psychoanalysts say that the symptoms the patients suffer from, symbolize their inner feelings. This may be true, but we need to understand that stress does not cause disease it only puts a burden on the weakest part of the body. Stress puts a burden on the body and makes it more susceptible to disease.

Some Symptoms of Emotional Stress

Symptoms of emotional stress include:

1. Situations seem worse than they really are.
2. Memory problems.
3. Concentration is difficult.
4. Negative thoughts
5. Very stubborn, feeling that everyone is out to get you.
6. Critical of everything.
7. Lose sense of humor, nothing seems funny.
8. Become demanding and want to control others.
9. Blame problems on others.
10. Escape is easier than coping.

Some Physical Symptoms of Stress

Symptoms of Physical stress include:

1. Stomach muscles tighten and may feel nauseas.

2. Heart rate increases. Anticipation of doing something you are afraid of.
3. Sweaty palms, perspire easily.
4. Shivering or trembling without being cold.
5. Tense muscles. Neck muscles tighten or between the shoulder blades.
6. Breathing patterns change.
7 Dry mouth, this happens to speakers who are nervous.
8. Physical feeling of fear.

It takes a considerable amount of time to change an attitude. And learning to relax is no exception. The first step is to recognize what factors interfere with relaxation. And secondly to consider what changes can be made to help with relaxation.

FOODS TO HELP THE NERVOUS SYSTEM

There are foods which can help build the nervous system. Fresh fruits are known to cleanse and nourish the body, including the nervous system. Fresh vegetables are full of nutrition and should be eaten daily. They contain properties rich in blood and bone building vitamins, minerals and enzymes. Whole grain products are very nourishing. Eat a variety including buckwheat, whole wheat, brown rice, millet, and corn meal. Herbal teas are relaxing on the body and can help reduce stress and nourish the body.

VITAMINS AND MINERALS TO HELP STRESS

Vitamin A is used up quickly when the body is under stress. It acts to sustain resistance to infection and repair tissue. It needs to be added to the diet when under stress.

The B-complex vitamins are all known to help with stress and the nervous system. All 17 related vitamins work together to perform many functions. They are needed daily to support and strengthen the nervous system. Pantothenic acid, a B-complex vitamin, is known as the antidepressant vitamin. It is thought to reduce anxiety and promote sleep. It is used to help build the body's ability to withstand stressful conditions.

Vitamin C stimulates adrenal function, protects vitamin E, calcium, hormones and enzymes from destruction and is considered an anti-toxin vitamin.

Calcium is needed in the nervous system. A lack may cause difficulties in concentrating. Calcium and magnesium help along with vitamin D.

Vitamin E protects the glands when under stress. It revitalizes the heart muscles.

HERBS TO HELP WITH STRESS

Some herbs thought to be useful to help the combat stress by strengthening the nervous system and relaxing the body include: alfalfa, chamomile, hops, kelp, lady's slipper, lobelia, mullein, passion flower, scullcap, suma, valerian, and wood betony.

AROMATHERAPY TO HELP STRESS

Orange blossom oil is thought to help ease problems associated with the nervous system and help with relaxation. It is also considered to help with insomnia.

Chamomile oil is known to contain calming properties. It is used as a mild nerve sedative and to promote relaxation.

COLOR THERAPY

The color blue is associated with relaxation. It is thought to ease the nervous system and relax the mind. It seems to soothe and promote a feeling of peace. Green is also suggested as a form of renewal and strength.

HOMEOPATHIC HELP FOR STRESS

Different homeopathic remedies are suggested to help with stress and strengthening the nervous system. Ignatia and magnesia carbonica are suggested as remedies in varying amounts and strengths according to the condition.

HYDROTHERAPY AND STRESS

Hydrotherapy is an easy method of relaxation. Alternating hot and then cold showers is thought to help. A hot bath in the evening before retiring is thought to promote relaxation and a restful sleep.

REFLOXOLOGY AND STRESS

In reflexology there are different areas of the feet associated with corresponding areas of the body. The areas of the feet related to the solar plexus, pituitary, and thyroid glands are suggested as areas to massage on a daily basis to help relieve stress and anxiety.

DIET

There are certain foods and products that are stressful on the body.

SUGAR

Sugar depletes the body of essential nutrients. It can wear the body down if consumed in excess.

CAFFEINE PRODUCTS

Coffee, cola drinks, tea, chocolate, and some medications all contain caffeine. Caffeine acts on the sympathetic nervous system. They are habit forming and mind-altering drugs. They interfere with relaxation often causing anxiety and fear. Eliminating caffeine products will aid in the relaxation process.

Ted Flicke, D.C., Ph.D., says in BESTWAYS magazine June 1986 page 58, "Caffeine acts directly upon muscles to increase their tension, stimulate the adrenal gland to produce adrenalin, and irritates the nervous system into unproductive, frantic activity. The physiological and biochemical events produce the universally recognized symptoms of caffeine - irritability, anxiety, nervousness, insomnia and inability to concentrate. Many victims of chronic stress related muscle tension find that their problems are completely resolved once caffeine is eliminated from the diet. "

TRANQUILIZERS

These are meant to alleviate stress. But they can deplete the body of nutrients and often cause side-effects. Tranquilizers can be very stressful on the body.

A diet rich in whole grains, fruits and vegetables is essential to a healthy body and mind. Eating processed foods, white sugar and flour, and caffeine products will eventually put stress on the body. Medical professional often emphasize the importance of eating healthy foods in abundance.

The B-complex vitamins are known as the anti-stress vitamins. All 17 B vitamins are interrelated. They fortify the nervous system. They are essential in helping the body to cope with stress. Vitamin A is used up quickly when and individual is under stress. It acts to sustain resistance to infections. It promotes growth and repair of body tissue. It also assists in maintaining normal glandular activity. Vitamin C stimulates adrenal function and is considered an antitoxin vitamin. Calcium is important for the nervous system. Magnesium often taken in combination with calcium is calming on the nervous system.

EXERCISE

Exercise is considered by many busy individuals to be a means of controlling stress and anxiety. Exercise can help to burn excess nervous energy helping to control emotions. A more physically fit and healthy individual can handle stress more effectively. Exercise can help benefit the body by increasing mental alertness and cognitive abilities, increase awareness, and aid in physical coordination. During exercise endorphins are released in the body which cause a feeling of well being. Many medical authorities are now recommending exercise as an antidote for nervous and emotional problems. Studies have shown that regular exercise is associated with increases in self esteem and decreases in depression.

NOISE

The sounds we hear have an immediate effect on the nervous system. Children crying certainly puts us on edge. And sirens make us tense. In contrast soft, soothing music can help us relax and calm our minds.

It isn't always possible to choose the noise we are surrounded by. When driving in traffic, horns honk, loud music and sometimes emergency vehicles are heard. But it is important whenever possible, to take time to relax with soft music or the peaceful sounds of nature.

TELEVISION

There are very few shows on television that actually promote relaxation. There is a lot of violence and stressful situations. Even the news is stressful. There are horrible incidents shown that occur each day. And hearing about them can make us concerned and anxious. Being informed is important. But don't be afraid to turn off the news. I have known children that have had nightmares from watching the news.

BREATHING THERAPY

Andrew Weil, M.D. in his book NATURAL HEALTH, NATURAL MEDICINE published by Houghton Mifflin Company, 1990 on page

117, suggests a breathing exercise used in yoga. He recommends it to his patients and considers this breathing technique to be a natural tranquilizer for the nervous system.

"Although you can do the exercise in any position, to learn it I suggest you do it seated with your back straight. Place the tip of your tongue against the ridge of tissue just behind your upper front teeth, and keep it there through the entire exercise. You will be exhaling through your mouth around your tongue; try pursing your lips slightly if this seems awkward.

First exhale completely through your mouth, making a whoosh sound.

Next close your mouth and inhale quietly through your nose to a mental count of four.

Next hold your breath for a count of seven.

Then exhale completely through your mouth, making a whoosh sound to a count of eight.

This is one breath. Now inhale again and repeat the cycle three more times for a total of four breaths."

It is suggested to inhale quietly through the nose and exhale audibly through the mouth. Andrew Weil suggest doing this twice a day for four breaths during the first month. Later is can be extended to eight breaths.

There should be a change in consciousness after the four breaths. This is a good response and is a sign that the involuntary nervous system is being affected and neutralizing stress. This can be used when confronted with a stressful situation as well as a technique to aid in relaxation and sleep inducer.

COMMUNICATION SKILLS

Learning to communicate and listen effectively are very important to reducing stress.

The heart rate and blood flow change during dialogue. As we speak, our blood pressure rises, and as we listen in a relaxed manner, our blood pressure is lowered.

Communication is a part of our world. It can give us a feeling of strength and support as we share with other the concerns we face and problems we encounter. And as we listen to others, we can encourage and support them.

Some other stress relieving techniques include yoga, meditation, and hypnotherapy.

Weight Control

Living in a nation where people are obsessed with dieting has lead to many different quick weight loss diets and programs. The media has stepped right in. Commercials are often seen offering easy methods to lose weight and become the person that you always wanted to be. We are constantly seeing individuals on television advertising products who are the perfect size and shape. And television and movie stars seem to always be slim and trim. Look where it has got them, wealth and fame. Some people are in constant battle with their bodies. Over weight people are often shunned or looked on with disapproval. Turning from one diet to another in order to develop the perfect size and shape which will lead to happiness for them. This obsession has lead to many of the eating disorders which plague our society. Anorexia nervosa and bulemia are common. And the female population especially think that their bodies must be perfect in order to be happy with themselves.

Dieting

But the problems with quick diet fixes is, they are not permanent. Studies have shown that weight lost quickly will almost always return. And unfortunately fad diets not only don't work and the weight is regained, but the body is more likely to gain back extra body fat with each diet tried. The only sure way to lose weight for the long term is a slow and gradual approach incorporating improved diet and exercise.

There is no miracle cure to the fat problem. Obesity can be controlled but not by taking a simple pill or supplement. And pounds will not be shed while eating a high fat diet.

Rapid Weight Loss

Rapid weight loss usually consists of water loss. And this will most definitely reappear. High protein diets cause the kidneys to work extra hard to remove the urea out of the body. And this leads to the water loss. Returning to a normal diet will lead to return of the water and weight. This type of diet is hard on the body especially the kidneys.

The most efficient and healthy way to lose weight is by concentrating on health and fitness. By changing the diet to a low fat, high complex carbohydrate diet with some protein, the weight will drop gradually. The changes need to be lifelong, and a commitment must be made. Add to this an aerobic exercise program and heath and fitness can be attained.

Modifying the Diet

Changes can be made gradually to a healthier lifestyle and eating habits. Concentrate on one step at a time. Learn to look for the fat content of foods and limit the fat intake. Add more whole grain products to the diet. Incorporate a variety of fruits and vegetables.

Recipes can be modified to fit with an effective diet. Choose recipes low in fat. Concentrate on using 10 to 20% of the calories in the form of fat. This would be approximately 13 to 30 grams of fat per day. Add whole grains to the recipe. Eat protein, sugar and salt only in moderate amounts.

1. Use light products in moderation because they still contain fat.
2. Use tuna in water instead of oil.
3. Substitute brown rice for white.
4. Check the fat content of products. Some spaghetti sauces are fat free or low in fat but taste the same. Or make your own.
5. Stick to white meat chicken.
6. Change to extra lean hamburger, rinse and drain before using.
7. Use olive or canola oil in moderation.
8. Use honey and apple juice concentrate instead of sugar.
9. When using eggs, for the most part throw away the yolk and use only the egg white. Instead of 3 eggs use 6 egg whites.
10. Use whole wheat flour in recipes to replace white flour.
11. Use white meat chicken, trim the fat, and remove the skin.
12. Make whole wheat pancakes for breakfast.
13. Use sugar free jams and jellies which are made using fruit juice with no added sugar.

14. Switch to 1% milk or skim milk.
15. Make your own oatmeal. The individual packages may contain large amounts of sugar.
16. Use 100% stone ground wheat bread.
17. Buy canned fruits in their own juice. Apple sauce is also available made without added sugar.
18. Stay away from diet or sugar free products that contain NutraSweet™. They are very stressful on the body.
19. Look for packaged cereals that are low in fat and sugar. Many are now fat and sugar free.
20. Use low fat yogurt in recipes to replace sour cream.
21. Use turkey breast and ground turkey in recipes requiring meat.
22. Eat lots of fresh vegetables and use a low fat dip.
23. Have plenty of fruit available for snacking.
24. Make home made muffins made with whole grains and little fat.
25. Use Molly McButter™ and cottage cheese on a baked potato.
26. Learn to enjoy the goodness of a healthy diet.

FOODS TO HELP WITH OBESITY

Food intake should be those which are associated with good health and nutrition. Fruits and vegetables should be eaten in abundance. Fresh and steamed vegetables provide vitamins and minerals. Fruit is considered a cleaner for the body and vegetables help build the body. High fiber foods are essential. Carrots, celery, beets and apple juice are thought to help stimulate and feed the glands. Lemon juice in a glass of water first thing in the morning is considered helpful for cleaning the liver and eliminating toxins from the body. Whole grains are good to provide fiber and enzymes to the body.

VITAMINS AND MINERALS TO AID WEIGHT LOSS

The B-complex vitamins are thought to help with appetite control and with the production of hydrochloric acid. This is known to aid in the digestion process. B_6 works with magnesium to break down proteins, fats, and carbohydrates. B_{12} aids the body in utilizing B_6, folic acid, and vitamin C. Vitamins A, C, and E help with the body metabolism. Iron aids the thyroid gland function.

HERBS TO HELP WITH WEIGHT LOSS

Some herbs thought to help with obesity and losing weight include cascara sagrada, dandelion, echinacea, fennel, kelp, papaya, parsley, and yarrow.

COLOR THERAPY

The color green is known to balance the system. It is thought that therapy using the color green may aid in restoring the balance of the body to help regain the proper weight of the body.

REFLEXOLOGY

To help with problems of underweight or overweight, the thyroid gland reflex areas of the feet should be massaged. Reflexes to the intestines can be massaged to relieve constipation sometimes associated with obesity.

A Table of 20 Common Herbs to Know

ALOE VERA (Aloe Spp.)

Aloe vera is a member of the lily family, though it looks much like a cactus plant. This plant is from Africa and grows in warm climates. It is easy to care for and great to have around. It requires little water and is hard to neglect. Kept on the window seal , it will thrive.

Skin Care

Aloe vera is very useful. It is known for its healing and soothing effect on burns, wounds, and rashes. It can help clean, soothe and relieve pain on contact. It is able to penetrate all three layers of the skin rapidly to promote healing. It contains salicylic acid and magnesium which work together to produce an aspirin like analgesic effect.

Aloe vera can be used to help prevent scarring and to heal minor scars. The properties of aloe vera help to promote healing as well as remove dead skin. It contains enzymes, saponins, hormones and amino acids which are absorbed through the skin. Aloe vera contains substances called uronic acids that are natural detoxicants and may take part in the healing process by stripping toxic materials of their harmful effects. The enzyme action is able to penetrate tissue and promote the healing and normal growth of the tissue.

To use the fresh aloe vera plant, cut off an outer leaf and split down the middle. Apply the gel directly to the burn or wound. The skin will soak up the gel and soothe the affected area.

Fresh plants are great to have around and without a green thumb I have found them easy to grow. Aloe vera products are available in health, natural food and drug stores. Many lotions are available containing aloe vera but may be present in very small amounts.

Aloe vera contains calcium, potassium, sodium, manganese, iron, lecithin and zinc.

ALFALFA (medicago sativa)

Alfalfa was used anciently as a miracle herb. The Arabs called it the "Father of Herbs."(Al-Fal-Fa) It has been cultivated for over 2000 years. In 400 B.C. the Medes and the Persians invaded Greece and began cultivating alfalfa there. They had brought it from the dry, hot regions of the Mediterranean where water was scarce. But Alfalfa is known for its survival. The roots of this plant can reach as far as 66 feet into the subsoil. The Romans discovered that alfalfa was excellent for their horses. The Moors took it to Spain and the Spaniards imported alfalfa to the new world.

RICH IN VITAMINS AND MINERALS

Alfalfa is a plant grown mainly for livestock feed. The United States is the largest producer of alfalfa. It is rich in vitamins and minerals. Alfalfa is considered to be perennial. It grows without being replanted for 5 to 12 years. Alfalfa is considered to improve the soil. There are over 50 species of Alfalfa in the world.

Alfalfa is thought to be able to remove poisons and the effects of poisons that may be in the body. It is also thought to neutralize the acidity of the body. Alfalfa is thought to break down carbon dioxide.

Alfalfa is considered by herbalists to be beneficial for many problems. And some recommend it for any ailment. It contains valuable minerals and vitamins which help assimilate protein, calcium, and other nutrients. It is thought to contain all the vitamins and minerals known to man. It also contains high levels of chlorophyll. Alfalfa is believed to be balanced for complete absorption by the body.

This excellent herb is recommended by herbalists for many different ailments including water retention, urinary and bowel problems, infection, muscle spasms, cramps, and digestive problems.

Alfalfa is rich in vitamins A, K, and D. It also contains the minerals calcium, phosphorus, iron, and potassium and some trace minerals.

BEE POLLEN

Though not actually an herb, Bee Pollen is rich in vitamins, minerals, protein, amino acids, hormones, and enzymes. In fact, it is considered to contain every chemical substance needed to maintain life. And thus, it is considered a complete food. Bee Pollen is a great supplement to build the immune system and provide energy for the entire body.

Bee Pollen is thought to have the ability to correct the body chemistry and eliminate unhealthy conditions. It is considered to have the ability to throw off poisons and toxic materials from the body.

Works with Body Chemistry

This valuable supplement is recommended for premature aging. It can help correct the body chemistry as well as metabolic imbalance.

Many use Bee Pollen as an immune system builder. It is full of nutritional properties and can help build the body. And athletes often use this supplement to help increase their strength, endurance, and speed. It is used as an energy booster.

Bee Pollen can help hay fever and allergy sufferers build up an immunity to irritating substances. This treatment is usually started in small doses. It is also thought to stimulate glands to promote a feeling of rejuvenation and boost the healing powers of the body.

Bee Pollen is rich in lecithin and increases the speed calories are burned within the body. It stabilizes poor metabolism which is often the cause of weight gain. It has therefore been successful in controlling and taking off weight by increasing the speed calories are burned. It is best taken by itself without food to help in correcting faulty metabolism.

Bee Pollen contains 35% protein. About half of this is in the form of free amino acids which are essential to life. It is also high in B-complex, and vitamins A,C,D, and E. It also contains Lecithin.

CAPSICUM OR CAYENNE (Capsicum frutescens)

Capsicum or Cayenne is considered by many herbalists to be a wonderful healer. It is found in a combination with other herbs because it seems to stimulate the action of those herbs. It is considered to be a general stimulant which allows this herb to increase the action of the body and organs.

CIRCULATORY SYSTEM

It is used to improve the function of the circulatory system and regulate the heart flow. It is also known to help normalize the blood pressure whether high or low. Capsicum is noted by many herbalists in the prevention of strokes and heart attacks because of its stimulation of the circulatory system. It is used for hemorrhaging both internal and external.

Capsicum was used in the past by herbalist treating severe cuts and even gunshot wounds. It was used externally and internally as a tea. Capsicum seems to have the ability to go immediately into the blood stream and adjust the blood pressure in the body. It seems to take the high blood pressure from a wound allowing it to clot and begin healing.

It is thought to have the ability to rebuild tissue and heal stomach and intestinal ulcerations. It is considered by some to be an internal disinfectant.

Capsicum is high in vitamins A and C. It also contains iron and calcium in high amounts.

CHAMOMILE
(Anthemis nobilis)

Chamomile is an herb which is recognized by many. It is considered to be a stimulant but is one of the best known nervine herbs. It is thought to be strengthening for the entire body.

CALMING EFFECT

It is commonly used for calming the nerves and as a sleep inducer. It is used by many in the form of an herbal tea. It is used as a sedative with no harmful side effects. Chamomile contains the amino acid tryptophan which works like a sedative in the body. Some herbalist recommend chamomile for hyperactive children.

It has been used to soothe an upset stomach and even for colic in babies. It has the ability to relieve indigestion and heartburn harmlessly. And Chamomile is thought to improve the appetite and aid in the digestion of food. It helps to eliminate gas and can work as a mild laxative. It can help to relax and calm the intestines.

Chamomile is thought to have a decontaminating effect on the toxins found in some forms of bacteria including staphylococcus and streptococcus. It may be able to ease colds and speed recovery.

It is thought to help regulate the menstrual flow and help with menstrual cramps by relaxing the uterine muscles.

Chamomile is high in calcium and magnesium which may be responsible for the soothing effect on the nervous system.

DANDELION (Taraxacum officinale)

This yellow weed commonly considered a nuisance growing in the lawn is a valuable herb. The entire dandelion is used including the leaves, flower, and roots. It is considered by herbalists to be a great blood purifier and can help individuals suffering from anemia.

My daughter opens the stem and rubs it on warts to remove them.

Dandelion is thought among herbalists to be beneficial on the functions of the liver. It seems to have the ability to clear toxins and obstructions and stimulate the liver.

SURVIVAL FOOD

This herb contains inulin which is a plant sugar and is beneficial to pancreatic action.

Dandelion is considered to be a great survival food. It is readily available and full of nutritional properties. It contains all the nutritive salts that the body uses to purify the blood.

Dandelion is beneficial for many ailments. It promotes healthy circulation, strengthens weak arteries, cleanses the skin, and can balance the gastric acids in individuals suffering from severe vomiting.

It is high in vitamins A, B, C, and E. It is also a natural source of protein. It contains potassium, calcium and sodium.

GARLIC (Allium sativum)

Garlic is considered by many to be a natural antibiotic. It is a powerful natural medicine as well as being a flavorful additive for many foods. It contains allicin, which is a natural antibiotic. It appears to be effective in fighting bacteria, viruses, and fungus. The properties of garlic seem to stimulate cell growth and activity. A study in Russia found that garlic had the ability to stop tumor growth in humans.

CHOLESTEROL

Garlic has been used to prevent and dissolve cholesterol in the bloodstream. It has the ability to open the blood vessels and reduce blood pressure in cases of hypertension.

For colds some herbalists recommend eating a clove of raw garlic. This seems to be effective in stopping the symptoms from the onset. The odor can be a problem. But eating parsley after the garlic, can help. The raw garlic contains the most antibiotic properties.

Garlic is thought to have a beneficial effect on all body functions. It is thought to stimulate the lymphatic system in ridding itself of toxins.

Garlic contains vitamins A, C, and B_1. It also contains selenium which is closely related to vitamin E in biological activity. Garlic also contains sulphur, calcium, manganese, copper, iron, potassium, and zinc.

GINGER (Zingiber offcinale)

Ginger root was an important economic item in ancient history. It was considered to be of great value. Greeks and Romans were using it as early as the first century A.D., and by the 11th century, it had become a common import from the Far East to the European market. In the middle ages it was used for medicinal purposes one of which was combating cholera.

Stomach Aid

Ginger has been studied and accepted as a remedy for an upset stomach. A study done a few years ago showed ginger to be just as effective as an over the counter medication in preventing and relieving motion sickness. Ginger is commonly used to soothe an upset stomach and indigestion. It is also used to ease the symptoms of the stomach flu. It can ease the complaints of nausea and vomiting. The resins in ginger are thought to be able to absorb toxic material in the stomach much the same as charcoal powder. It can aid in the digestion process.

It is also thought to aid the respiratory system. Herbalists recommend ginger for fighting off colds and flu, removing congestion, clearing a sore throat, and relieving aches and pains. It has also been used for cleansing the bowels and kidney.

Ginger has been used often in combination with other herbs. This is thought to enhance their effectiveness. For instance, ginger and capsicum are used together for bronchial congestion.

When used as a hot tea, ginger can induce perspiration. It seems to act as a general tonic for the body. The pioneers used this herb as a stimulant and for heart palpitations and fevers.

Ginger contains protein, vitamins A, C and B complex. It also contains calcium, phosphorus, iron, sodium, potassium and magnesium.

GOLDEN SEAL (Hydrastis canadensis)

Many herbalists consider Golden Seal to be one of the most important members of the herbal kingdom. It is usually found in every herbal medicine chest. It grows wild in the eastern sections of North America. But because of its popularity, it is now being cultivated.

Healing Herb

Golden Seal is used as a healing herb. It is known for its antibiotic properties. It is thought to contain antibiotic and antiseptic properties which can help fight staph and strep infections. The active ingredients of golden seal contain hydrastine and berberine which are strong antibiotics. Golden seal is thought to heal quickly and effectively. It does not need to be taken for long periods of time. Small doses over short periods of time are recommended.

It is recommend by herbalists to boost a sluggish glandular system. It may help regulate the liver function. It is used for congestion in the nose, bronchial tubes, throat, intestines, and stomach. It is thought to have the ability to heal mucous membranes in the body and is considered to be a general medicinal herb.

Golden Seal can be used as an antiseptic to clean boils, wounds, and ulcers. It can also be used as an eye wash. It should be strained before being put in the eye.

Some herbalists recommend the use of golden seal for people suffering from diabetes. It seems to provide the body with nutrients which act like natural insulin. It helps the body to regulate the mechanism to allow the correct use of sugar. It has been found effective in reducing excess blood sugar. Some people have been able to gradually eliminate insulin while slowly adding golden seal.

This valuable herb is recognized as a stimulating herb which can invigorate and strengthen the body.

Golden seal contains vitamins A, C, B complex, E, and F. It contains calcium, copper, potassium, phosphorous, manganese, iron, zinc, and sodium.

HOPS
(Humulus lupulus)

Hops is found commonly throughout the world. It was originally used as a food. The tips were cooked and eaten. The young plants were eaten because the older were too tough. The North American Indians used hops for medicinal purposes including aches, pains, and insomnia.

SEDATIVE

Hops is recognized as a natural sedative in the herbal community. It is known by many as one of the best nervines in the herbal kingdom. It seems to be strong but safe to use. Its main uses are to alleviate nervous tension and promote a restful sleep. It has been used to relieve insomnia naturally.

A poultice of hops is recommended for inflammation, boils, tumors, and swelling.

Hops has been used as a stimulant to the glands and muscles of the stomach and also as a relaxant on the gastric nerves. It also has a relaxing influence upon the liver and gall duct and a laxative effect on the bowels.

Hops is rich in vitamins B-complex and C. It contains magnesium, phosphorus, potassium, zinc, copper, traces of iodine, manganese, iron, sodium, lead, flourine, and chlorine.

KELP
(Fucus versiculosus)

Kelp is known for its natural iodine content. This natural plant iodine is absorbed slowly and safely by the body. Iodine is essential in the body to aid in the function of the thyroid gland as well as the lymph glands. The lymph glands aid in building the body's immunity against infection. And the thyroid gland is responsible for metabolism, energy and proper growth. Kelp is also useful for stimulating all glands of the body. Iodine is necessary to prevent goiter, emotional problems, and in brain function.

GLANDS

Kelp is recommended for boosting glandular health including the thyroid, pituitary and the adrenals. It has the reputation of speeding up the burning of excess calories by increasing the body's metabolism.

Kelp is thought to be beneficial on many disorders of the body. It is considered to be a valuable supplement to build and maintain a healthy body and mind. It is used to aid the nervous system and the brain function normally. It is often taken during pregnancy because of its rich abundance of minerals.

Kelp is thought to have a binding effect on the liver to eliminate toxins as well as supply minerals for normal function. The liver is sensitive and works continually to clean toxins from the body and kelp helps strengthen the liver to perform its function. It also has a beneficial effect on the colon, bladder, and kidneys.

Kelp is considered to be strengthening on the heart. It seems to naturally clean the arteries of build up.

It contains almost all the minerals considered vital to health including iodine, calcium, sulphur, and silicon. It is rich in B-complex vitamins, A, C, and E.

LICORICE (Glycyrrhiza glabra)

Licorice is considered to be a natural source of the female hormone estrogen. It is used for female problems with the reproductive system.

It works as a stimulant on the adrenal glands. And it is thought to be a natural source of a hormone similar to cortisone.Licorice is thought to stimulate the production of cortin hormone which helps when coping with stressful situations.

It has also been known to help with lung, throat, and chest complaints. Licorice contains glycosides which have the ability of purging excess fluid from the lungs, throat and body. The saponin content is thought to be responsible for the expectorant action. It has the ability to loosen the phlegm in the respiratory tract and help the body expel the mucus. It has a reputation of being effective in relieving coughs. It is also an important herb when recovering from illness because of its ability to supply energy to the system.

LAXATIVE

Licorice is also known for its laxative effect and in helping heal inflammations of the intestinal tract including ulcers. It is useful as a mild laxative for children because of the mild taste. It has been used for gastric ulcers.

This herb is thought to help control cholesterol and maintain healthy arteries. It is also used as a blood cleanser along with other herbs.

Licorice contains vitamin E, B-complex, biotin, niacin, and pantothenic acid. It also contains phosphorus, lecithin, manganese, iodine, chromium, and zinc.

LOBELIA

RELAXANT

Lobelia is known by herbalists for its ability to relax the entire body. It seems to work quickly and should be used only in small doses but does not seem to have any harmful effects. Lobelia is considered to be the most powerful relaxant in the herbal kingdom. It is thought to have the ability to relax muscle fiber and alleviate spasms.

It is thought to have the ability to remove disease and promote healing in the body. It seems to have the ability to remove congestion from the body including the blood vessels.

It is used for croup and respiratory problems. Lobelia is thought to be especially useful in relieving bronchial spasms. It is recommended for bronchial problems and pulmonary complaints. It seems to work quickly to remove mucus.

Lobelia is recommended for many uses including pain. Herbalists use the extract on aches and pains by massaging the Lobelia on sore muscles.

Lobelia has been used externally in a poultice with Slippery Elm to bring abscesses or boils to a head.

Lobelia contains sulphur, iron, cobalt, selenium, sodium, copper, and lead.

MULLEIN (Verbascum thapsus)

Mullein has a long history. It was used by the Greeks and Romans for many ailments.

The Europeans used the roots for coughs and cramps. It was used for all lung ailments. The American Indians used mullein as a basic remedy for sprains as well as lung problems.

Mullein is an herb which seems to contain some narcotic properties without being habit forming. It is used as a pain killer and a sleep inducer. It seems to calm the nervous system.

EXPECTORANT

It is considered an expectorant herb. It can aid in controlling coughs, cramps and spasms. It seems to soothe inflamed and irritated tissue. It is also thought to loosen mucus and move it out of the body. It seems to be valuable for all lung problems because it nourishes as well as strengthens. It seems to irritate the lining of the bronchioles to stimulate the expulsion of mucus and relax and soothe bronchial spasms. Mullein's action to loosen and eliminate mucus out of the body is important when the lungs are congested. The sooner the congestion is cleared, the less chance of infection. It is beneficial for asthma and emphysema and infections involving the upper respiratory system. It is helpful for chronic coughing and smoker's cough.

Mullein is thought to protect irritated or inflamed tissue. It is used to reduce irritation in the bowels and digestive system. It is used to prevent diarrhea and soothe digestive muscle spasms.

Mullein has been used for many ailments including warts, dropsy, sinusitis, swollen joints, tumors, sore throat, and tonsillitis.

Mullein is high in iron, magnesium, potassium and sulphur, It also contains vitamins A,D, and B-complex.

PARSLEY (Petroselinum sativum)

Parsley is a common herb found in the local supermarket. It is often used as a preventative herb. It seems to have the ability to increase the body's resistance to infection and disease. Some herbalists even recommend Parsley to be used as a cancer preventative. They say that Parsley contains a substance in which cancerous cells are unable to multiply.

Parsley is often used as a natural diuretic. It is better on the body than drugs used as diuretics because it will not deplete the body of the necessary potassium. It is recommended for kidney and bladder problems.

This herb is used to help digestion. It is present in the green drink used by many people because of its nutritious properties.

Parsley is suggested as a means of regulating the menstrual cycle. It can also help with other female complaints. It can help dry up the milk in nursing mothers. And for this reason, it is not recommended for mothers nursing their babies. It is also thought to help alleviate the after pains of childbirth.

Unlike most herbs, every part of the parsley can be used. This includes the plant, roots, leaves and seeds.

PREVENTATIVE

Parlsey is a good preventive herb. It contains vitamins and minerals and is rich in chlorophyll. It contains easily assimilated vitamin A that helps feed the glands to regulate the hormone output. It is high in iron which is beneficial in strengthening the liver.

Parsley is recommended for many uses including increasing resistance to infection and disease, strengthening the muscles, healing the urinary tract, and as a digestive aid.

Parsley contains vitamins B, A, and C. It is high in chlorophyll and iron. It contains some sodium, copper, thiamine, riboflavin, silicon, sulphur, calcium and cobalt.

PEPPERMINT (Mentha piperita)

Peppermint is used throughout the world as a medicinal plant. It is cultivated in Europe, some parts of the United States, Australia, and the Orient. It grows wild in the eastern United States. Peppermint was brought over with the colonists as a medicinal herb.

The menthol in peppermint is responsible for the herbs beneficial properties. The oil of the peppermint contains about 50 to 78 percent menthol. Menthol acts as a stimulant for the flow of bile to the stomach which aids digestion. It also acts as an antispasmodic, calming the digestive muscles.

Peppermint is often used to make a mild tea. It can be used hot or as a chilled tea in the summer. It is used primarily to soothe the stomach and help with digestive problems. It can help alleviate colic, stomach pains from indigestion, diarrhea, colitis, and ulcers. It also works as a sedative on the stomach and to help strengthen the bowels.

STRENGTHEN THE BODY

Peppermint is also know for its effects as a nerve stimulant. It is thought to clean and strengthen the entire body. It is used as a general relaxant. And it is also thought to strengthen the heart muscles. The stimulating effect of the peppermint brings oxygen into the blood stream.

This herb is thought by herbalists to help with many problems which include mental fatigue, throat infections, senility, viruses, headaches, pain, arthritis pain, dizziness, hysteria, vomiting, and menstrual cramps.

Peppermint contains vitamins A and C. It contains many minerals including magnesium, potassium, inositol, niacin, copper, iodine, silicon, iron, and sulphur.

RED RASPBERRY (Rubys idaeus)

FEMALE CONCERNS

Red Raspberry is considered an excellent herb for many female problems. It is thought to contain nutrients to strengthen the uterus wall and the entire reproductive system. It seems to aid in morning sickness, prevent hemorrhage, and reduce the pain in childbirth. It can be used throughout pregnancy and labor. Some herbalists use this herb as a tea to relieve painful menstruation and decrease the flow. It is also used to help enrich the colostrum found in breast milk.

The Red Raspberry tea is mild and pleasant to the taste. It is mild enough for children as well as adults.

It can be used for children with colds, diarrhea, colic and fevers. It is soothing to the stomach and digestive system.

Red Raspberry contains vitamins A, C, D, E, G, F, and B. It contains the minerals iron, phosphorus, manganese, and calcium.

SENNA (Cassia autifolia)

LAXATIVE

Senna is known in the herbal community as a laxative because of its ability to increase the peristaltic movement in the intestines. It is thought to have a strong laxative effect on the entire intestinal tract including the colon and large intestines. It is not recommended when there is an inflammation in the stomach or intestines because it may cause irritation. It should be taken with ginger to prevent cramps.

Senna is also recommended for ridding and eliminating worms and parasites from the colon.

It can be used with all illnesses to cleanse the system. And it has the ability to tone and restore the digestive system as it cleans.

SLIPPERY ELM

Slippery Elm is thought to have the ability to neutralize stomach acidity and to absorb foul gases. It can aid in the digestion of milk and other foods the body has difficulty digesting. It can help soothe irritations and inflammations of the mucous membranes. It is useful whenever there is a problem digesting food.

HEALING

It is considered by herbalists to assist the adrenal glands and in healing the body. It seems to help stimulate the output of the cortin hormone. This helps send blood building substances through the system.

Slippery Elm is thought by many to draw out impurities and heal all parts of the body. It is used as a remedy for ailments of the respiratory system. It seems to be able to remove mucus from the body.

Slippery Elm contains vitamins E, F, K and P. It also contains iron, sodium, calcium, selenium, iodine, copper, zinc,. potassium and phosphorus.

YUCCA (Yucca glauca)

Yucca is a common plant found in the desert regions of the Southwest. It is a relative to the cactus family and a member of the lily family. The plants are beautiful and many desert regions use the yucca to decorate their yards.

The Indians used the root of the plant to cure skin problems and ulcerations. It was used on the skin to stop the bleeding from cuts and to reduce the inflammation from injuries. The roots of the Yucca plant were also used as a poultice on breaks and sprains.

ARTHRITIS

The Yucca plant has a high content of the steroid saponins. These are similar to cortisone. For this reason, the Yucca is beneficial for individuals suffering from arthritis and rheumatism. Some believe that the Yucca saponins improve the body's ability to produce its own natural cortisone by supplying the materials needed for it to be manufactured by the adrenal glands.

Yucca is thought to strengthen the intestinal flora. It is used to aid in the digestion of food by keeping the wrong type of bacteria out of the digestive tract. It helps to break down accumulations of undigested waste that can collect in the colon..

Yucca is used in sewage treatment plants throughout the United States to break down organic waste more rapidly.

Yucca is used for many ailments including high blood pressure, lowering cholesterol, headaches, and arthritis.

The root of the Yucca plant contains a high amount of vitamins A and B-complex and some vitamin C. It is high in calcium, potassium, phosphorus, iron, manganese, and copper.

Bibliography

Bamer, Donald R., B.S., D.C. APPLIED IRIDOLOGY AND HERBOLOGY. Provo, Utah: Woodland Books, 1982.

Bieler, Henry G., M.D. FOOD IS YOUR BEST MEDICINE. New York: Ballantine Books, 1965.

Blauer, Stephen. THE JUICING BOOK. Garden City Park, New York: Avery Publishing Group Inc., 1998.

Calbom, Cherie and Maureen Kean. JUICING FOR LIFE. Garden City Park, New York: Avery Publishing Group Inc., 1992.

Carter, Mildred. BODY REFLEXOLOGY. West Nyack, New York: Parker Publishing Company.

Colbin, Annemarie. FOOD AND HEALING. New York: Packet Books, 1990.

Colgan, Michael, M.D. YOUR PERSONAL VITAMIN PROFILE. New York: Quill, 1982

Cooper, Kenneth H., M.D., M.P.H. AEROBICS. New York: Bantam Books, 1968.

Cooper, Robert K., Ph.D. HEALTH AND FITNESS EXCELLENCE. Boston: Houghton Mifflin Company, 1989.

Griffin, LaDean. THE ESSENTIALS OF IRIDOLOGY. Provo, Utah: Woodland Books, 1984.

Hainer, Cathy. "Aromatherapy wafts into mainstream science, business." USA TODAY, 1 July 1992, sec. D, p. 6.

Hausman, Patricia and Judith Benn Hurley. THE HEALING FOODS. Emmaus, Pennsylvania: Rodale Press, 1989.

Jensen, Dr. Bernard. FOODS THAT HEAL. Garden City Park, New York: Avery Publishing Group Inc., 1988.

Kaye, Anna and Don C. Matchan. REFLEXOLOGY FOR GOOD HEALTH. No. Hollywood: Wilshire Book Company, 1978.

Lieberman, Shari, M.A., R.D. and Nancy Bruning. DESIGN YOUR OWN VITAMIN AND MINERAL PROGRAM. New York: Doubleday and Company, Inc., 1987.

Lieberman, Shari, M.A., R.D. and Nancy Bruning. THE REAL VITAMIN AND MINERAL BOOK. Garden City Park, New York: Avery Publishing Group Inc., 1990.

Lust, John, N.D. and Michael Tierra, C.A., O.M.D. THE NATURAL REMEDY BIBLE. New York: Pocket Books, 1990.

Maclvor, Virginia and Sandra LaForest. VIBRATIONS. York Beach, Maine: Samuel Weiser, Inc., 1979.

McCarthy, Paul. "Exercise and the Big C." AMERICAN HEALTH, March 1992, p. 121.

Null, Gary and Shelly Null. THE JOY OF JUICING. New York: Golden Health Publishing, 1992.

Ott, John N. LIGHT RADIATION AND YOU. Old Greenwich, Connecticut: The Devin-Adair Company, 1982.

Ritchason, Jack. THE LITTLE HERB ENCYCLOPEDIA. Provo, Utah Woodland Books, 1982.

Ritchason, Jack. THE VITAMIN AND HEALTH ENCYCLOPEDIA. Provo, Utah: Woodland Books, 1986.

Tenney, Louise, M.H. HEALTH HANDBOOK. Provo, Utah: Woodland Books, 1987.

Tenney Louise, NUTRITIONAL GUIDE WITH FOOD COMBINATIONS. Provo, Utah: Woodland Books, 1991.

Tenney, Louise. TODAY'S HERBAL HEALTH. Provo, Utah: Woodland Books, 1983.

Tisserand, Robert B., THE ART OF AROMATHERAPY. New York: Inner Traditions International Ltd., 1979.

Toufexis, Anastasia. "The New Scoop on Vitamins." TIME MAGAZINE, 6 April 1992, pp 54-59.

Weil, Andrew, M.D. NATURAL HEALTH, NATURAL MEDICINE. Boston: Houghton Mifflin Company, 1990.

Index